a leg up

josh sundquist

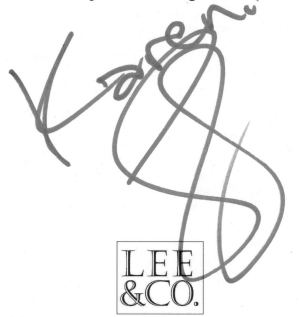

LEE
&CO.

A Leg Up

Published by Lee&Co.
1550 Hunting Avenue
McLean, VA 22102
LeeAndCoBooks.com

Please note that as of the publication date of this book, the author's marital status is still classified as single. All interested applicants may submit spousal requests to the aforementioned address.

International Standard Book Number 978-0-9802097-2-3
Library of Congress Control Number 2008900075

Columns from *The Richmond Times Dispatch* and *The Newsstreak* reprinted by permission

contents

becoming a speaker

sarcastic observations

training for 2006

sweet bonus columns

end matter

intro

Dear Esteemed Reader,

Let me begin by congratulating you on your high level of intelligence and wherewithal* as evidenced by your purchase of my book.

A Leg Up is a collection of stories that I wrote as a columnist for both the *Richmond Times Dispatch* and *The Newsstreak*, my high school newspaper. I selected my favorite columns through the years and arranged them in loosely chronological order for this book.

What will you read about in *A Leg Up*? There are several stories about my battle with cancer and my amputation. And since I wrote most of these columns as a teenager, many are about my years as a novice ski racer, inexperienced motivational speaker, and generally girlfriendless-loser.

You might say this is an autobiography about growing up. Enjoy.

-Josh

---

* I am not entirely sure what this word means

life through rose colored goggles

Originally published in *The Newsstreak*

Ever since I lost my leg to cancer, I've always tried to focus on what I *can* do. But realistically, there are limitations. There are things that no matter how positive I feel or how courageous my spirit happens to be that day, I will never be able to do.

Back when I was a kid, and everyone played baseball, I would hit, and someone else would be my "runner." Sometimes my runner would eventually make it around the bases and score, and people would high-five me. I really didn't have much to do with it. Sorry.

That's why I was so excited the first time my Mom told me about "adaptive skiing." She said that a group of kids from the hospital were going to Massanutten to learn to ski, and I was invited to go along. The first time I put on skis, I remember being amazed by how heavy they were, but also by how smoothly they could slide. By lunch time, I could ski faster than I ever could've run with two legs.

My Mom has always said that I got into skiing because I liked to go fast. I guess maybe she's right. I like fast food, fast facts, and fast music, but I hate corn on the cob. (It just takes too long to eat). I loved that first season—progressing to the top of the mountain, coming down fast and feeling the wind blow through my stocking cap on my shiny head. For a few moments, I could forget about having one leg.

When the snow started to get slushy and my lift ticket was about to expire, I would go inside to find my parents in the ski lodge. We had the system all worked out: They would take off my stocking cap, and I would quickly replace it with a baseball cap, worn backwards to hide the balding effects of the chemotherapy.

I'd go home and become a cancer victim and hospital patient again. I'd lie awake at night in the hospital, watching the chemotherapy dripping into my veins. Drip, drip, drip. I wanted to rip out all the tubes and get back to the mountain. I dreamed of being free again, being "able" again. Sometimes I dreamed of racing. I'd heard rumors about a "U.S. Disabled Ski Team," that would let people like me go to the Olympics. It would be awesome to do something like that someday, I thought. With that, I would close my eyes and begin to dream.

chemotherapy, skiing just don't mix

Originally published in *The Newsstreak*

Chemotherapy and skiing are a lot like those water and oil demonstrations you see in science class. You can shake them together all you want, but they just don't mix. Besides taking your hair, chemotherapy zaps your energy, your time and your health.

That first season I skied three times. By the end of the second day, my instructor had taken me on the hardest trails on the mountain. I was happy – or at least for a while. Then I realized what I really wanted: to compete. I wanted to be able to go out and give my all, to do my absolute best, and most importantly, to win. I was very excited to learn that my local mountain actually had a ski race for disabled skiers at the end of the season. I could compete!

In that first race, I really had to concentrate. "Left on blue, right on red, left on blue, right on red," I said to myself, trying to follow the correct path through the ski gates. After the race, when they announced that I had won the division of one-legged juniors, I felt surge of victory. I had done it. But as I walked up to receive my medal, I noticed that I was the *only* one-legged junior. Of course I won.

As I sat through the rest of the awards, I realized that every single skier got some kind of medal. Even if the category had to be something ultra-specific (you know, like "Most Improved Blind Skier Whose First Name Starts with an 'S'"), everyone got an award. Suddenly the race seemed less like a competition and more like one of those elementary school science fairs where everyone wins a "Certificate of Participation." In other words, it was not a real competition.

But after the award ceremony, an elderly man approached me.

"I used to coach the U.S. Disabled Ski Team," he said. "I think you've got a lot of potential."

we need to be prepared for game time

Originally published in *The Richmond Times Dispatch*

She looked down at her clipboard and then up at me, and then at the clipboard again. "Follow me, please," she said. My parents and I followed her down a short hallway inside Disney's MGM Studio One.

The lady with the clipboard brought us into a room and sat us down on some couches.

"We thought we'd give you and Steve some time to get to know each other before you go on," she said.

She shut the door, and left the four of us in a room. My parents, me, and Steve Young, the Superbowl MVP quarterback of the San Francisco 49ers. This was five years ago, I was just eleven years old at the time, so I don't remember much about what was said. But there we were, Steve Young and I "getting to know each other."

A few minutes later, Steve and I were escorted to the studio floor. Someone handed us two bottles of spring water and sat us down in those folding canvas chairs that movie directors use. In about two hours, we'd be on prime-time national TV.

Taken before a few cameras, we rehearsed our four-minute segment. He asked me a little about how I'd just learned to ski, and I talked about how important it was that people call up now and give to their local hospital.

"Thirty years ago, people with my type of cancer wouldn't have had a chance," I said.

After the practice, my Dad and I went to find some food in another part of the building. On the way back to the studio, we passed some make-up rooms. The door to one opened, and out walked Mike Kryzewski, a.k.a. "Coach K," the man who has led the Duke Blue Devils to two national championships.

"Hi, Josh!"

How'd he know my name?

"I saw the practice hour of the broadcast," he said, answering my question before I asked it. "You did great!"

"Thanks, I'm pretty nervous," I confessed.

I know we've all heard of great, inspirational comments from important people. But it's very rare that they hit home in applying to something in our life. What Coach K told me next has been one of those things that I know I will never forget because not only was it brilliant, but it applied perfectly to what I was dealing with.

"I'm gonna tell you what I tell my players," he said. "When someone plays well in practice, I know that they can be awesome when it comes to game time, because they can use the excitement of the game to help them play better than they ever could've in practice. Josh, you did awesome in practice. You'll be incredible when you're on the real thing."

To this day, I like watching a few minutes of the Blue Devils on TV. Not really because I want to see the basketball passed around the court, but to see Coach K, wincing at a missed foul shot, pointing at a player, drinking Gatorade and everything else that a coach does. And when I see him, I remember what he taught me about life, and about game time.

I believe that every person in this world will have their own game time. It can come in many forms. A chance to testify to someone's innocence in court, the opportunity to pull a child from the bottom of the pool and perform CPR, or being there to smile at a stranger who believes there is no hope left in life.

I am as guilty as any high schooler of wishing that I could be living in a constant game right now, one that doesn't involve classes and homework and SATs. But the reality is that Steve Young didn't wake up one morning and try out for the NFL. To have the opportunity to be a top notch game time performer, he spent hours, weeks, years…practicing. And then, when he caught the snap and looked out towards the receiver, he used the excitement of the game to be able to throw the ball farther than he ever could in practice.

I don't know when my game time will be. I don't know what it will look like. What I do know is that I want to be ready. I want to have practiced enough excellence and enthusiasm towards life that I can make a big impact with whatever I do. As for now, I am content to prepare for life and believe that I can go far at game time.

how I live with a disability

Originally published in *The Newsstreak*

I'm fourteen years old. It's been five years since my amputation. I've heard most of the questions by now, and I've developed mostly standard answers.

"What happened to your leg?"

"I had cancer."

"Are you better now?"

"Yeah."

"What's your fake leg made out of?"

"An aluminum skeleton covered with soft foam and rubber skin."

But sometimes I get caught off guard. A girl named Eboni surprised me last summer with a question I'd never heard. Looking at my leg, she asked, "Is the foot fake, too?"

"No, actually they managed to sew my real foot back onto the end of the leg," I said. After Eboni thought about what she had just asked, we both laughed till we had tears in out eyes.

I'll never forget that.

I've heard many good questions. But I can always tell people are afraid to ask me substantive questions because they are afraid of how I might answer. What if I don't like to talk about it? What if I hate having a disability and I will take my anger out on them?

Whenever I am around kids, it's obvious that this fear is learned at a later age. When kids see me with my artificial leg off, they usually make a subtle sign that they have noticed. It comes in the form of the child screaming, "Mommy, that boy's leg fell off!" I've had kids who keep looking at me from different angles by walking circles around me, trying to figure out where my other leg is.

Last year I discovered that kids in Mexico are just as curious. The only difference is, I had absolutely no idea what they were asking me. I was, however able to guess that they were wondering about my leg when I heard the word "uno." My typical response was, "Quatro anos en el pasado. Tengo cancer, pero ahora yo bien." This translates to something like, "Four years in the past. I have cancer but now I good." One of two things always happens after a kid notices my disability. Sometimes I get the chance to explain, "My leg was sick, and the doctors had to cut it off." Unfortunately, more then often than not, the kid's Mom jerks the kid away with, "Haven't I told you never to stare?" or "What made you ask a stupid question like that?"

The problem is that I know what will happen next time the kid sees someone who's "different." People like me should not be stared at or talked to. I'm someone who must be feared, because I hold a secret that will remain a mystery.

If the parents would let their kids ask questions, of course I would tell them. I don't want them to think that I shouldn't be noticed since I'm disabled. They need to see disabled people in a good light, because sooner or later they will have to learn a lesson the hard way: Many people limp through life, but only God notices. That is, we all have disabilities, and some are less obvious than others.

The saddest reality for people who are different is that sometimes fear can make others hurt them deeply. I have been fortunate in that I can only remember one time I was directly made fun of. It was during my first week at Boy Scout Camp.

I had finished chemotherapy just six weeks before, and my hair was finally growing back. Being only ten, I was afraid of what people might think about my disability, so I wore my artificial leg for the whole week. Despite my efforts, some boys found out about my leg during the "First Year Camper's" program. I don't know why, but one of the boys began calling me a "stupid handicapped kid." It hurt me, but I didn't know what to do, so I tried to ignore him. But some of the guys from my troop refused to ignore this kid. Later that day, we were building towers out of long wooden poles. My friend Finney "accidentally" laid him out with a pole to his head.

Somehow my parents knew what had happened when I got home. I remembered the exact way my Dad brought it up.

"I heard about the stupid kid who called you handicapped," he said.

He told me that it is true, I am handicapped. There's nothing wrong with that. But people that think that I am less of a person because of my handicap are stupid themselves.

At the time, I thought it was a typical father's corny play on words. But looking back, I have realized the truth in what he said. I can't deny that I'm different. That is reality, and not accepting it would be setting up myself for disappointment.

Everyone has disabilities. We all have differences. And each day, we all can choose how we want to respond to those circumstances.

cancer survivor now celebrates life

Originally published in *The Richmond Times Dispatch*

"Smoking or non?" asked the greeter in Ruby Tuesday's lobby.

"Non-smoking, please," Shawn said.

As we sat down in our booth, Shawn grinned at me.

"I can't imagine anyone who's had cancer wanting to be in smoking," he said.

I nodded a polite agreement and mumbled something to the affirmative, trying not to be impressed that he had thrust into the core of my being before we'd even ordered drinks.

Soon, our waiter came and explained how hard it was coming back from vacation and returning to work. I felt almost enough sympathy to make a mental note to give a twenty percent tip, but then I realized I wasn't paying. Shawn was taking me out to dinner, to hang out and "shoot the bull," as he likes to say. I have met lots of other cancer survivors, but usually they are pretty old. Shawn is in his late twenties.

He was nice enough to order an appetizer, Ruby Tuesday's own "Super Sampler." As I munched fried potato skins and hot wings, something inside me warned that too much fat can cause heart disease. People who have had cancer should wait for their salad.

After Shawn gave me some advice about college, we discussed hobbies. Sailing is his favorite, but he also likes the high adventure stuff and wants to try sky diving.

a leg up

"I like do things like that, because cancer has taught me to live life to the fullest," he said. "We don't know how much longer we have to live, and it's important to do everything you can, because life is an incredible gift."

I wanted to raise my hand and remind him that I, too, am a cancer survivor. But I let him continue reflecting my personal philosophies.

"People get depressed, [and] I just want to shake some sense into them," Shawn said.

In his words, I could hear myself.

These things, I knew, are what I think of every day – from the moment I wake up to when I fall asleep. These things drive me to value my time like a lost explorer holding his last piece of bread. I see people wandering aimlessly through their short lives, and it pushes me to speak and write about this moment we call life.

While Shawn continued his commentary, I thought of the days when I've awakened upset about something trivial – a test, lack of sleep or a cold. It is a crime infinitely worse than eating fried potato skins. Then I smiled and reminded myself that most days, I jump out of bed, put my hand on my chest and rejoice that I am alive. I hop over to the mirror and praise God that I can still stand on one leg. I love to look in the mirror and notice that I have hair – that I don't have to select a baseball cap to cover the bald head that sat on my neck during chemotherapy.

After we waited for our waiter to return from his smoking break, Shawn paid the bill and we took a walk through the mall.

We compared the chances of survival that our doctors had given us. Compared with my fifty percent, he was a walking miracle at three percent. Of course, I had cancer just five years ago, but he was diagnosed back in the '80s – before many medical advances.

A few weeks later, I'm back at school, walking around on a brand new artificial leg. The people there, at school, can't understand why I'm so happy to be alive. Maybe I should call Shawn.

in scouting/life, joy is in the journey

Originally published in *The Richmond Times Dispatch*

"Joshua, if you were to get lost out in the woods overnight, you'd probably die."

This less-than-inspiring phrase was the parting wisdom from my Dad when I left for my first Boy Scout camping trip. It was also the phrase that was playing incessantly inside my head the following evening, prompting me to shout things like "HELP!" and "Somebody save me!" at ever-increasing decibels.

As a new Scout at the ripe age of eleven—and a relatively new amputee of one year—I had made the mistake of wearing my artificial leg on an orienteering course set out for our troop. (Orienteering can be summed up in three words: map, compass, woods). To make a long story short, I made it through about half of the course to find myself in waist-high bushes that left my artificial leg and me rather immobile.

After two hours of tears, whistle blows and replays of my Dad's ominous parting words, a band of rescuers from my troop found me stuck in the bushes on top of a ridge. Scoutmaster Mr. Graham hoisted me onto his back, and he and the highest ranking Scout in our troop "evacuated" me from the area.

Upon returning to the campsite, no one believed that I was indeed stuck—not *lost*, big difference—and to this day I am occasionally called upon to defend my orienteering skills among my fellow Scouts.

a leg up

Last week I attended a friend's Eagle Scout Ceremony, and it prompted me to think back on my own time in the Scouts. I have many memories—some good, some bad—but all hard-earned life stories that will stick with me forever. Like "Camporees," which are events where multiple troops gather to burn things and play with dangerously sharp pocket knives. A few years back, at the New Market Camporee, we were going to sleep in our tents at night when a storm brought a sudden wind burst at 85 mph, followed by torrential rain and the kind of lightning where you hear the thunder before you can even get out the "one" in "one-one-thousand." As my tent-mate and I held up the roof of our badly mangled tent during the storm, we were quite convinced that we were facing our last moments on earth. (My tent-mate was crying, actually, but I kept that secret between us to shield him from eternal cry-baby status in our troop).

Or how could I forget the induction weekend to Order of the Arrow, Boy Scout's camping honor society? I'm now sworn to secrecy about what's involved with the "Ordeal" required for membership, but I will tell you several things that the weekend does not involve: food, shelter and/or speaking.

Back in my early Scouting days, I spent several hours a day on my merit badges. I was a true Scout Nerd, on track to earn my Eagle Scout rank by age thirteen. I will never forget a particular Board of Review I had with my Scoutmaster to discuss my fast ascension through the ranks.

"Josh," he said, folding his big hands and setting them down on the conference table, "I feel like I could put you in a room with a list of all the tasks required for Eagle, and you would come out a few hours later with all the work done."

"OK," I said, accepting what I perceived to be a compliment.

"No, that's not the point of Scouting," he said. "It's about the experience. It's about coming in as a boy and coming out a few years later as a man. You gain skills and knowledge. You mature."

There was a long pause in our conversation. I had never considered Scouting in this light. To me, it had always been a checklist of achievement, a map to a certain success called "Eagle Scout."

"OK," I said after some time, nodding my head with a certain added understanding.

I left that Board of Review with a different perspective on my weekly meetings and monthly camping trips. Scouting was a journey, not just a destination, and the joy was in the journey, not just in wearing a certain badge.

I did get my Eagle at the age of thirteen, but I didn't immediately quit as I had originally planned to do. I stayed on for a while, leading and providing an example to the younger Scouts. Because after all, life is a journey, not a destination, and the joy is in the journey, and in bringing others with you on the trail.

mission trip puts present in perspective
Originally published in *The Richmond Times Dispatch*

When I first met Luis almost two years ago during a mission trip, it was so dark I could barely see him sitting in his wheelchair. He was staring at a tiny black and white television – a luxury in the slums of Mexico City.

We entered the room, which had cinder-block walls and a dirt floor, and sat down. The first few awkward moments redefined my idea of small talk. I know very little Spanish and Luis knew absolutely no English.

My Dad and a guy named Dan had joined me on this visit to Luis's house. They know Spanish, so they could talk to him. I have one leg, so I was supposed to be able to "relate" to him. Our mission was to persuade Luis to attend a Bible camp that a church across the street was planning with the help of people from my church, including Dad, Dan and me.

During our translated conversation, I told Luis I would understand if he didn't want to participate in all the camp activities, but we would help him with anything he wanted to do. After some thought, he agreed to come. The next day an old bus pulled into the neighborhood. Luis wheeled down the sidewalk with his Mom. She came to remind us to be careful with her seventeen-year-old son. His degenerative bone disease made him very fragile.

We took the bus to a place a few hours outside the city. After unloading, we played soccer and capture the flag. Luis just watched. And he saw me, the disabled guy who was supposed to be able to sympathize with him, running around on my forearm crutches and playing soccer, just like the other kids.

Luis gradually opened up. He started to laugh more and sometimes contributed to the discussion during Bible study. After a few days of watching the other kids in the pool, Luis decided that he wanted to try swimming. With lots of help from the counselors, he got in and floated around, smiling the whole time.

Unfortunately, all good things must come to an end. After about a week, the old bus showed up and took us back to Mexico City. For Luis, this meant it was back to sitting in a wheelchair in a dark room with a dirt floor and a little black and white television. It was sad to see him go back to this immobile lifestyle, but there was nothing we really could do. After eleven days in Mexico City, my church's mission team piled back into that same old bus. This time, it took us to a modern airport with running water, air conditioning and fast food.

Last spring (almost a year after our return to the United States), the pastor of the church that we worked with in Mexico called my Dad with news about Luis. Ever since our trip, Luis had changed. He started going to church and Bible studies. He smiled more and laughed a lot. But positive attitude can do only so much if you are a wheelchair-user in Mexico City. Unless something changed, Luis wasn't going anywhere besides the church across the street. Fortunately, that's what this phone call was about. Luis wanted change.

Ever since our visit, he had wanted to try forearm crutches – just like mine. But there was no place to buy them. The pastor knew that my Dad was returning to Mexico the next summer to work at Vacation Bible School, and he wondered if we could help.

My Mom called Walk Easy, the company that makes my crutches, and explained the situation. A few days later, a brand new pair of bright red crutches arrived in the mail, free of charge. My Dad took them to Mexico and dropped them off at Luis's house.

A few days passed, and there was no news from Luis. Then one day, while my Dad was at his host family's home, which was several blocks from Luis', there was a knock at the door. In walked Luis, using his new crutches and smiling.

Nine months have passed since Luis got his crutches, and I haven't thought much about him. But a couple of weeks ago, I was running a few laps around the block with one leg and forearm crutches. For a few minutes, I wondered what it would be like to run with two legs, fast and free. Then I remembered a guy in the dark room, sitting in a wheelchair on a dirt floor. He was grateful to even have crutches.

life lessons from Jones Soda

Originally published in *The Newsstreak*

Being a fan of Jones Soda, I have discovered that even a soda bottle has a lot to say about life.

1. **Life is best when we celebrate differences.** One of the unique things about Jones Soda is the labels. In the words of the bottle, "they're always changing." The labels on Jones soda are always different, often weird (like the picture of the two drunk ladies), but I've noticed one thing in observing my fellow Jones drinkers. No one ever complains about the different bottles. In fact, just the opposite. We enjoy the weird photos on our bottles. We "celebrate" them. In the same way, people are all different, sometimes weird. You have a choice in each of your relationships. You can either discriminate based on differences, or celebrate them.

2. **Life is interactive.** The labels on Jones bottles come from customers who send them in. Chances are, if you send them a unique photo, you'll eventually find it on a Jones. It's an interactive soda. Guess what else? It's an interactive life. You reap what you sow. You get out what you put in. Remember the Golden Rule?

3. **Minds are like bottle caps.** If you keep them closed all the time, you're screwed. (It's a pun, get it?) The lesson is obvious. I don't know anyone who buys a Jones and leaves the cap on. If you never open the bottle, you can't enjoy the soda! And when you can't

open your mind long enough to listen to other points of view, you're not enjoying life like you can.

4. **Your fortune is on the inside.** Frequent Jones drinkers know to always look inside their bottle for a fortune. Under the cap of every Jones is a fortune. Kind of like in a fortune cookie, but not always as profound. My favorite Jones fortune is, "Before you criticize someone, walk a mile in their shoes." The moral of the story is that in your life, just like in Jones, your fortune is on the inside. You could look great, be a smooth talker and be a fashion model and not get anywhere in life if you didn't remember the inner you is just as important. Thus, in your life, your real fortune is on the inside.

5. **Appearances can be deceiving.** As you can see in my photo, Jones Soda bottles have the same shape as a kind of bottle that I can't legally buy for another six years. When drinking Jones, I am always questioned by concerned citizens as to whether I am drinking alcohol. I guess the appearance of the bottle is kind of deceiving. But just like the concerned citizens, we sometimes assume the worst about someone based on appearances.

6. **Sheetz is a great place.** As the only Jones retailer in my city, Harrisonburg, you have to give them some credit as a convenience store. Not only do they have cheap gas, but great food, a cool intercom, and good coffee.

7. **If a company tries to sell 12 oz. they will have a good image. If a company tries to sell a good image, they'll need to produce a lot more than 12 oz.** On Jones' web site (www.JonesSoda.com), the company philosophy quotes *The Wall Street Journal*, October 9, 1995, "The beverage industry is more about image than taste…" Urban Juice, Jones' owner, concentrates on creating a dynamic, popular image

that can be sold easily to our generation. They believe in doing this, sales will follow. In other words, who cares what Sprite says? Image is everything.

8.   **One person with a great idea can change history.** At school, my friend Ben was the first Jones drinker. He bought his first bottle over a year ago. After Ben drank that first Jones, he told some of his friends, and they told some more people, until now, a lot of students can identify it. Many people's knowledge of Jones can be tracked to Ben. So what do Buddha, Martin Luther King, Jr., Jesus Christ and Ben have in common? They all had a good idea, and changed history with it.

9.   **Quality is never cheap.** My parents don't seem to understand why I spend a dollar for only 12 ounces of soda. The answer is simple: it's the best soda available, and the best isn't cheap. Yeah, it might take a few extra quarters, but I say it's worth it. A lot of people think they can take shortcuts on their way to success. In terms of soda, shortcuts are called "Value Choice" and "Simply Soda." Thomas Edison, founder of General Electric and inventor of the light bulb, put it well. He said, "Genius is one percent inspiration, and ninety-nine percent perspiration."

10.   **Life is fragile.** A glass Jones Soda bottle seems pretty solid doesn't it? But we've all seen what happens when glass is dropped. It breaks very easily. Even though glass is fragile, Jones keeps putting their soda in glass, not aluminum, because glass is special. Just like glass, life is precious and fragile. Having cancer at the age of nine taught me some important lessons. I learned that even the best of us aren't invincible. One hundred years from now we'll all be gone. Seize the day.

car trouble shortens personal connection

Originally published in *The Richmond Times Dispatch*

I have an annual tradition of missing the Rockingham County Fair.

I do this because almost anything is more fun than looking at livestock, collecting brochures and riding a Ferris wheel.

But this past summer, on August 16, I had two good reasons to attend. The first was a concert. The second was a girl.

The concert featured Jars of Clay. I spent the hour with other teens trying to find a place where security wouldn't catch us moshing. After the show, I finally talked to Lydia. The girl.

I approached her at the right time. Fifteen years old and without a license, she was looking for a way home. I smugly jingled my keys.

"I can take you home," I said.

After a long pause, she agreed to let me give her a ride if I would take her friend Meredith, too. I agreed.

For a while, we wandered around looking at livestock, and for some reason, I found myself enjoying the animals and their smells. But we looked at animals so long that this 16-year-old began to worry about his 11:30 p.m. curfew.

So I suggested we leave. This took a long time because most of the guys at the fair either knew Lydia, thought they knew Lydia, or wanted to know Lydia.

Every few steps, Lydia would be embraced by another excited male fairgoer. She'd introduce us and I would casually mention that I was giving her a ride home. This earned me many jealous looks.

It took a good twenty minutes to get out of the fair. Finally, I thought, I could talk to her.

When we got to my car, I spent several proud moments showing Lydia and Meredith the new bumper stickers and license plates on my 1983 Toyota Camry. I climbed into the driver's seat, and they both got in the back. (This was the first sign that my night was doomed). Then I switched on my headlights.

Nothing happened.

I looked out the window to be sure, and they were definitely not on. In this dreadful millisecond, I felt my fantasies of a happy car ride home together evaporating along with my drained battery.

Still hoping, I turned the key several times. All remained quiet in my car.

"I left my lights on," I said, reminding myself to breathe.

Before I knew what was happening, Lydia and Meredith burst out the back door and ran off into the distance. I remained in the car, moaning softly and bouncing my head on the steering wheel.

There I was, on the tenth day of my life as a 16-year-old. I'd always told myself I'd date at this age, but now I wanted to put it off for a few more decades.

I looked across the parking field to see Lydia and Meredith hop into a sports car that soon drove toward me. Great, I thought. They've come to mock me as they drive off with someone who owns a decent car.

Instead, the car stopped quickly, and three ultra-cool dudes got out. Lydia and Meredith followed. Their leader, the owner of the car, eyed my Toyota suspiciously.

"Yeah, I can jump his car," he mumbled.

Cool Dude No. 2 grabbed some jumper cables from the back, and in no time, our hoods were up. I soon discovered that despite the swagger with which No. 2 was carrying the jumper cables, he had no idea what he was doing. He clipped the cables in various combinations on our engines until the owner of the sports car was satisfied. Then he started his car.

"Turn the key!" Cool Dude No. 3 yelled at me. I did and nothing happened.

"You have to rev your engine," No. 3 yelled to his friend behind the wheel.

The owner of the car was quite pleased with this suggestion. Soon, he was revving his engine like petroleum was going out of style, and continued to do so long after being instructed to stop.

Finally, a middle-aged woman heard the commotion and came over to help. She instructed us to match "red with red." Cool Dude No.2 nodded. "Oh," he said. "Red with red." When I turned the key, my car started.

While we waited for my battery to stabilize, Meredith and the owner of the sports car flagged down a security guy on a golf cart—they wanted to borrow his pen to exchange numbers.

Twenty long minutes later, I pulled into Lydia's driveway.

"Um, maybe I will call you sometime," she said as they climbed out of the car.

"Yeah," I said, trying to fake enthusiasm.

A few weeks later, I drove by myself to another concert. Meredith and the guy with the sports car were there, holding hands. (His name is Tyler, it turns out). We talked for a few minutes and I thanked him again for the jump.

I didn't bother to ask about Lydia.

mourning a friend who battled cancer

Originally published in *The Richmond Times-Dispatch*

The news came in an e-mail. It was a note from Jennifer, a girl I know from a camp for kids with cancer that we both attended. At the end of her e-mail, she made a strange comment.

"I took the news about Levi pretty hard."

"What news?" I replied, pretending that I didn't know the instant I read the e-mail. I knew all too well what it meant when a sentence had the word "news" and a fellow cancer victim's name in it.

After sending my reply, I started to think about Levi. I usually saw him a few times a year, at which time he would greet me with an engaging "S'up, dawg?" I have a clear image of Levi balancing his right crutch with his left hand while he slapped me a right-handed five.

In the beginning, Levi and I seemed so similar. We both battled through endless chemotherapy treatments and hospital stays. After we both lost a leg to cancer, it seemed as if we had won our lives back.

At cancer camp and teen cancer weekends, Levi and I often played soccer. We both loved it. Although I played a lot before my amputation, I think soccer is the middle name of everyone in Levi's family. He even wore soccer gloves (I guess they helped him grip his crutches better).

We did our best to keep up with everyone on the soccer field. When we were on the same team – both stuck back on defense – we would discuss our one-legged soccer moves. When we were on opposing teams, we'd argue about whether hitting the ball with a crutch counted as a handball or not. And is it a penalty when you trip someone with your crutch?

Last winter, I saw Levi at a teen cancer ski weekend. His hair was thin, almost gone. I knew what that meant. Relapse. Levi's cancer had returned. Unfortunately, we didn't ski together much because we were at different ability levels. Mostly, I watched him from the lift. He would ski a little and fall. Ski and fall. Ski and fall. I hated to see Levi fall.

I wonder what he thought when he saw me hitting jumps, trying to get big air. I wonder if he was hurt that I didn't ski with him more, or try and help him up when he fell. I hope not. I don't know, I hope that maybe my skiing was an encouragement to him. I don't know, and I will never know.

Levi always lived with a sense of destiny. I remember a talk we had at cancer camp in August. I learned that the cancer had relapsed in seven tumors in his lungs. Not a good diagnosis.

"Now I just keep getting as many surgeries as I can…"

His voice trailed off and he looked away. I nodded.

"Do you smoke?" he asked a few minutes later.

"No," I said. "Do you?"

"Yeah. It's kind of relaxing, you know?"

Actually, I didn't know, and I wanted to scream at him for doing something that would damage his fatally diseased lungs, but I cut myself short. I didn't know what he was going through. I fought a tough battle, but I never relapsed. Levi was going through something I couldn't understand, and it wouldn't be right for me to judge him.

Levi was a smart guy, though. He knew smoking was bad for his lungs. One thing was for sure: If he was smoking, he had given up hope.

For cancer patients, giving up hope is the last battle. And being terminal means you have to lose. I hated to see Levi lose.

The dreaded "news" would come sooner or later, and it eventually came in Jennifer's e-mail. Levi died December 2. He was fifteen and a sophomore at Lancaster High School in Lively.

We were so similar. We were so much alike. But now, more than five years after we were first diagnosed, here I am, alive and healthy, while Levi is dead. Life isn't fair, and it isn't certain. Only death is certain. But seeing how I am still alive, I guess my mission here isn't finished yet. I have work left to do. And if you're reading this, I guess your mission isn't complete, either.

I sure wish Levi was reading this, too.

wheelchair games changes view on life
Originally published in *The Richmond Times Dispatch*

Usually when I go to the pool, everyone else has two legs. People always stare at me. I am the abnormal one.

So I wasn't surprised when people stared at me during the swimming competition of the Mid-Atlantic Wheelchair Games held at Harrisonburg's James Madison University last month. The difference was, none of the swimmers there had legs. Normally when I go to the pool, I have to hop to get around and everyone feels sorry for me. Sometimes they tell me how difficult it must be to have to do things with one leg.

But at the games, for the first time in my life, I actually felt a little guilty hopping around the pool. Just being able to use one leg set me apart as a person who had it pretty easy. There I was, effortlessly hopping around, while the other competitors got out of their wheelchairs and crawled into the water.

Sometimes, when I swim laps at the gym, I get annoyed because kicking with one leg doesn't make for a very fast stroke. (In fact, without concentration, kicking with one leg can make you swim in circles.)

At the games, I was the only one who could kick. This advantage became quite obvious when I swam in the same heat as the teen-age wheelchair-bound competitors. (Our times were not compared.)

"Oh, no!" they said when I got in the water. "You're gonna lap us!"

I'd tried to laugh and downplay it.

"I'm not that fast," I said. "Don't worry."

"Yeah, but you can kick!"

I couldn't deny that.

Sure enough, I lapped them.

Come to think of it, I don't even know why the officials let non-wheelchair-bound athletes compete in the games. But they did, and I'm glad.

The next day I went to the track events, this time just to watch. As the competitors raced around the track in their brightly colored team shirts and "racing chairs," I noticed that the coaches and parents were constantly yelling at them to "push, push, push." Of course, this is a normal phrase to hear at a track meet, but it occurred to me that pushing is not just a metaphor in wheelchair racing. Pushing is the way the competitors move.

They seemed really fast and I was curious just how fast. Using my artificial leg, I walked over to a little trailer where two women were scribbling down the results.

"What's the national record for Juniors in the mile?" I asked.

"It's Matt Barber. He's here today...three minutes and forty-eight seconds," said one woman of the record Matt set in 1999 – in the sixteen to eighteen-year-old group competing at the next to highest level. It has yet to be broken.

Wow.

One thing is for sure: That's certainly a lot faster than I could hope to go on my crutches. On the other hand, on my crutches, I can go up and down stairs, I can run through a field and I can hike up a mountain.

With my one leg, I can jump on the trampoline and I can ride my bike.

My eight-year old brother, Luke, said it well while we were watching some of the swimming events.

"Josh, at least you still have one leg," he said.

In fact, driving to the swimming events and seeing all the handicapped parking spaces filled up by the guys who had to crawl into the pool taught me something. It made me wonder why I am even allowed to use handicapped spaces.

I really don't need them. I am blessed enough that I can park anywhere. So at the games, I parked my car in the farthest corner of the lot, just because I could.

in life, timing is everything

Originally published in *The Richmond Times Dispatch*

I have a nice routine for exercising. It's challenging, it's simple and it kills the time that I might otherwise spend worrying about ill health.

A few weeks ago, while I was enjoying a typical high-speed, high-perspiration bike ride, I noticed something unusual. I was short of breath. Not the kind of shortness of breath you experience when you bike really fast and you have to rest, but a kind that made me feel as if I was only inflating my lungs to half-capacity.

I dismissed the problem, however, so I could spend the rest of the ride daydreaming about my plans for the distant future. I imagined myself in 10, 20, 30, and 40 years, never stopping to consider whether I would actually live that long. Besides, how could I have a medical problem? I work out every day!

The following week, I kept exercising and I kept having difficulty breathing. But even with the continued problems, I didn't have time to go to the doctor. It was exam week, besides, I had speaking engagements, writing deadlines and phone calls. Lots of phone calls. I certainly didn't have time to go to the doctor's office.

Still, getting out of breath is kind of annoying. One afternoon I decided to make sure my exercise was easy, so I went for a walk. But to my dismay, each step brought me more shortness of breath and more worry. At home a few hours later, I was even having trouble breathing while sitting still.

Sitting there, struggling to breathe, I recalled a chemotherapy drug that doctors gave me six years earlier. This drug is known to damage the heart.

"If you have any symptoms of heart failure, such as shortness of breath, I need to know immediately," my doctor always said.

This memory prompted more symptoms. I felt nauseated, light headed, and my arms started to hurt.

"Mom, I'm scared."

As my parents got on the phone with the doctor, I couldn't believe what was happening. I had always known that death could be around the corner. I had always known that life, as the Bible says, "is like a vapor." But now I was being caught by surprise.

I feared the knowledge that my life could end that very night – just like that – and the world would go on spinning the same number of feet per second. As usual.

Suddenly, the minutes before me turned into gold, as precious as every second of my sixteen years had been. I sat down at the computer and frantically attempted to finish a book I had been working on for several months. I briefly instructed my Dad on how to get it published. That night, I was determined to make certain that the vapor of my life left at least a droplet to run into the future.

As the seconds continued to slip away, I realized that somewhere out there, a timer is counting down my life. Obviously, God hides the timer from human view. But that night, it was as if I could see the furthermost digits, which count the seconds and tenths-of-seconds. I will never know how much time I really have left, but by remembering the timer's smaller numbers – the seconds and tenths-of-seconds – I know that time is passing, and it's passing fast.

attitude changed by national tragedy

Written September 11, 2001. Published in *The Richmond Times Dispatch*

There was something about the color guard. Maybe its members' shoes weren't quite as shiny as they could have been, or maybe their march was a little out of time. Maybe it was something about the way they presented the American flag. The flag seemed to them, and definitely to me, just another everyday part of life at Fort Mead, Maryland.

It wasn't that the flag didn't hold power. It held an incredible power, and maybe that was the problem. Maybe America had become so strong that we took our power for granted. But when they presented the colors at 8:30 a.m. this morning, we were still living at a time when nothing could touch the American flag.

Fifteen minutes later, the time when it all started, our breakfast was being served. We ate our food and began the program promptly, because timing is always perfect on a military base.

Several minutes later, I confidently approached the podium and began my speech. This was certainly not my first time speaking at a charitable fund-raiser, and I was sure it would go off without a hitch. Like the flag erected behind me, I couldn't be touched.

Pride, as they say, goes before the fall. Even as I delivered the first line of my speech, a cell phone rang. The recipient of the call became very serious and left the room. As I kept speaking about making a difference, cell phones kept ringing and people kept walking out.

While I spoke, a colonel in the audience kept looking down at his pager. No matter how hard I concentrated on my delivery, he just kept looking at his pager, often turning to confer with another highly decorated soldier to his left. I felt helpless and confused. My speeches had always interested and captivated the audiences. Why wouldn't they listen to me?

I delivered my final line, and the audience clapped for eight seconds. The event's host then approached the podium and waited for everyone's full attention. Fourteen seconds later, there was a collective gasp. No one could believe what had happened. The woman to my right grabbed my hand and began to cry.

"Help us, Jesus," she whispered.

Within fifteen minutes, I was stuck on the beltway with thousands of other cars that were trying to evacuate the Washington, D.C. area. The most powerful government in the world had been shut down. As I circled the city en route to Virginia, the traffic jam trickled past the Potomac River. From that position, I could look in my rear view mirror and see the Capitol building. The Washington Monument was to my right. Even though it was standing as tall and proud as ever, it was dwarfed by the gigantic cloud of smoke billowing up over the Pentagon.

As helicopters and fighter jets whizzed in the air, I drove beneath an overpass where a man and a woman were holding an American flag. They just stood there, holding that beautiful piece of cloth and casting small shadows on the interstate. They seemed so sad, so touched.

I, too, had been touched. But I was only touched emotionally. My life was not torn apart as the lives of so many thousands had been just a few hours earlier.

When America woke up on the morning of September 11, it woke up with the "it-can't-happen-here" attitude that had been built over several decades of peace and prosperity. It had been a slow process, much like the little specks of dirt and oil smears that build up on a color guard member's dress shoes after too many routine presentations.

But maybe this tragedy will force us to wake up with a different feeling. Maybe we can wipe off our shoes and march in unison again. Maybe America can step up to a new level of strength, thus warding off more tragedies.

Timing on a military base, after all, is always perfect.

live now, not later

Originally published in *The Richmond Times Dispatch*

At the age of six, my greatest joy and fulfillment came from a game I called "Boys vs. Girls." The major premise was that each gender was united in opposition against the other. Each also wanted to demonstrate its superiority.

At first, we boys believed that running around the playground yelling catch-phrases about the supremacy of males contributed to our victory. Then, a few of us decided that an even better way to "win" the game was to kiss the girls. With this discovery, we concentrated all of our resources on the important and difficult task of kissing.

I actually had some success in this mission, and it was this victory that earned me the title "Kisser" from every girl on the playground. One of the recipients of my forced affection apparently was flattered, and she began passing me love notes in swimming class. (I had to smuggle them under my shirt so as to stay undiscovered).

Eleven year later, I can see that when it comes to dating, I haven't fared as well. I've only had one girlfriend, and that was a middle school relationship that blossomed for twenty-three hours before I got dumped.

Last year, there was a girl named Lydia. After I jump-started our relationship by leaving my car's headlights on—and thus running down the battery—while we went to the fair, she stopped showing up for our dates. She stood me up six times before I got the message. (Girls are just so subtle about whether they like you.)

The following summer, I asked a girl named Amy to go golfing at a par-three golf course. About halfway through the nine holes, I made a particularly good shot. But, in my ecstatic celebration, the knee on my artificial leg buckled and I fell to the ground.

Amy tried to act sympathetic without laughing, but when I stood up, I discovered a major problem: The foot on my artificial leg had turned around the wrong way. (This aroused many worried looks from the other golfers.) I spent the remaining holes banging my foot into trees in hopes of getting it back in the right direction.

I often recall the moment when I lay on the golf course green with my foot turned the wrong way. I could've felt sorry for myself. After all, it was our first date, and how many first dates do you get? But I chose instead to laugh. Why? Because it was our first date, and why should I let it be ruined by a little problem?

I want to live life like that little boy running around the playground trying to kiss girls because he thought it would somehow help prove the superiority of his gender. I want to give a cheerful wave to any driver who flips me the bird because I don't have time to sit around letting other people ruin the way I feel.

perm a catalyst for making change
Originally published in *The Richmond Times-Dispatch*

If you're a guy and you're at Wal-Mart buying a box labeled "Seven Day Perm," you're going to get some weird looks. Believe me, I know.

And yes, the perm was for me. It was Spirit Week at school, the time when you're actually allowed to break the dress code, and doing so somehow bolsters school spirit. Instead of breaking out the old food-coloring-in-the-hair trick for "Crazy Hair Day," I opted for a temporary perm. I got the aforementioned kit at Wal-Mart and had a female friend apply the chemicals. The next morning I arrived at school with my freshly curled hair poufed up in a fro. (And yes, I even put a pick in it).

Over the next several days, I surveyed my hair carefully for signs that the perm was disappearing. Since I'd bought a "Seven Day Perm," I figured it would only last three or four days. Let's be honest here: We all expect to get what we pay for.

It's the scarcity mentality. For example, if I decided to give you a Christmas present, you could expect me to spend on you what you'd probably spend on me, if not less. After all, since when would anyone get more than he or she gave?

Anyway, back to the story. A week passed, and my bleached-blond hair still retained a distinct likeness to Ramen Noodles. That is, it still looked like it did the day it was curled. And, unfortunately, my hair's newfound undulation did not go unnoticed. I lost count of the number of times I had this conversation:

"Ummmm, Josh?"

"Yeah."

"Did you get a … perm?"

"Well, …sort of."

On my first Sunday at church as a curly haired Christian, I received so many quizzical glances that I skipped Sunday School and went directly home.

As the weeks passed, my friends began asking me the obvious question: How permanent, exactly, was this Seven Day Perm? In fact, as I write this column, my so-called "seven day perm" has retained its effect on my hair for exactly 67 days. My friends now badger me with accusations that I attend daily "re-perming" sessions at the beauty salon. Some friends.

What all this mayhem has shown me is that, sometimes, you get more than you pay for. In this case, the perm kit cost $7, so I was expecting to pay $1 per day for a seven-day perm. Instead, I paid $7 for a 67 day perm. (Note: While these extra two months have been nice, I would've preferred that Wal-Mart simply write me a check for $60 for the 60 additional days).

Since it's possible to get more than you pay for, I figured the reverse also must be true. And if Wal-Mart can do it for me, why can't I do it for other people? What I mean is, there's nothing wrong with giving more than I expect to get. In fact, maybe it's good thing.

After all, anyone can get a good grade by doing what's required, but you can earn an A+ only by doing more. The need for staying alive might be fulfilled with junk food, but you can be more healthy by eating right and exercising. You might be able to get by in your relationships by loving just enough, but why not "do unto others" and give more?

Oh yeah, if you were on my Christmas list this year, you may have noticed that—unlike last year—your gift didn't come from the "Everything's $0.99 or Less" store.

making a bid for the U.S. ski team

Originally published in *The Richmond Times-Dispatch*

I looked at the other guys around the breakfast table. I knew that we all wanted to make the U.S. Disabled Ski Team. That was why we skied, why we raced and why we came to this Christmas Race Camp in Colorado.

True as that was, however, we didn't discuss our goals. It doesn't take a genius to figure out that there are only so many spots on the U.S. team, and only the best make it.

For those 10 days, we slept, ate and skied at Winter Park Ski Resort. But that morning, we ate earlier than usual because we were supposed to meet with Paul Dibello before we hit the slopes. We knew that Paul, as director of Winter Park's disabled program, can influence who makes the U.S. team.

The other skiers and I wondered what he would say. Would he invite us back? Would he tell us to get a life and find a regular sport? In short, the tension at breakfast was thicker than my instant oatmeal.

At 8:30 sharp, we walked to Paul's office.

"One at a time, please," he said from behind his desk.

John went in first. John and I are both teens with one leg, but he's been racing for five or six years. In fact, out of the five teen-agers at the camp, I was the only one with virtually no racing experience (although this is my sixth year skiing). Add to this the fact that we were training with "full-time" disabled racers, who had moved to Colorado from around the world, and you can see why the coaches nicknamed me "rooksta."

While we waited for Paul to finish talking to John, I looked at a group photo of the U.S. Disabled Ski Team on the wall. I wondered how it would feel if my face were in that photo.

John walked out of the office.

"Any bruises?" someone whispered.

"Next."

I volunteered and walked in.

In the corner of Paul's office were his "ski legs." When Paul skies, he apparently takes off his two artificial legs and puts on his ski legs, which are mounted in ski boots. I wondered whether those were the same ski legs he wore during his 12 years on the U.S. Disabled Ski Team.

"How do you like race camp?" he asked.

"It's awesome."

(I found out about the camp when I called Paul in November to get information about a race at Winter Park. He could sense my excitement about racing and invited me to Christmas Camp.)

"You think disabled racing is something you want to get into?"

"Yeah, definitely."

"People have been saying good stuff about you," he said.

"Oh, yeah?"

"Yeah. The coaches say that you have a lot of raw talent. Maybe even more than some of the other people here."

Paul nodded toward the hall where the more experienced racers waited. Then he paused.

"Do you want to be on the U.S. Team?" he asked.

This was a question I was ready for. I looked him straight in the eye.

"Heck yeah!"

"It's gonna take you five years of training," he said.

I knew I could do it in less than five years, and Paul knew it, too. I also knew this was a test. Paul was challenging my desire.

"OK," I answered blankly.

"Well, maybe only three years."

Apparently, I had passed the test.

"But it's gonna take a lot of work," he continued. "You're gonna have to be an animal out there. You're gonna have to train like crazy and go in the gym to get big."

Another challenge.

"You would move out here and go to high school in the morning and then be here to train in the afternoon."

"I might be interested," I said.

"It would mean leaving your high school your senior year."

"I know," I said.

Paul was testing me again, trying to get me to back down from a challenge.

"I bet you have a lot of friends back in Virginia."

This was enough testing for today.

"Look, there are some things that are important," I said. "And then there are goals."

Paul understood. Being a member of the U.S. Disabled Ski Team is my goal, and I'm willing to make some short-term sacrifices for the long term pay-off.

Several weeks later, I think "sacrifices" might not be a strong enough word. First, I will have to convince my parents that I'm ready. Then I will have to give up my friends, my school and my security to transfer to a new school in the middle of the Rockies. To top it off, I will need to raise at least $15,000.

Sounds like another challenge.

headed to Colorado to train for a medal

Originally published in *The Richmond Times-Dispatch*

I dream of the day when someone will see the sticker on my car and say, "Oh, are you a fan of the U.S. Disabled Ski Team?"

"I'm on it," I will reply.

I want to be the best one-legged skier in the world.

I want to change peoples' perceptions of disabled skiing from "Isn't it swell that the gimps went out to ski" to "Those guys can rip with the best of 'em!"

I want kids with two legs to see pictures of disabled skiers in the sports section and say, "I want to be that good."

Most of all, I want the thrill of competition.

I used to play Little League Baseball and soccer. I was good at both, but I dreamed of being the best. Then, at age 9, I lost my leg to cancer, and my dreams of victory shrank to hopes of participation.

By the time I was a freshman at Harrisonburg High School, I had been deprived of real competition for four years. So I joined the wrestling team. It was tough; I barely made it through practice every day. But I kept on, focusing daily on how it would feel to win.

Despite my effort, I got pinned in every single match (usually in the first minute). This was no competition. It was a thrashing, plain and simple. So I decided to concentrate on skiing, and this year I joined the Massanutten Ski Team. I've been practicing often and working out almost every day. I even found a used racing suit.

I've been in three races. In all three, my times have been dead last. The only people I can beat are the skiers who disqualify by falling or missing a gate. This tells me one thing: I need to practice. A lot. Like every day, at the best facility in the country for disabled skiers. That would be in Winter Park, Colorado, where most of the U.S. Disabled Ski Team and its aspiring members train.

I used to think that I could move there some time later, maybe after college, or at least after high school. Then I took a trip out there and learned that the other 16-year-old guys with one leg are already faster than me.

I learned something else in Colorado. Those guys—my competitors for a place on the U.S. Disabled Ski Team—are still in high school (like me), and they don't want to give up their comfortable high school for skiing. So most of them are still racing part time while they finish school, and just training a couple days per year. I say, bring it on. Hit me hard. I say it's time for me to jump out of my comfort zone. I say it's time to be the best.

I've decided to move to Colorado next year for about four months, from January to April. I would go to a local high school every day until noon and then drive to Winter Park to train for a few hours. As a part of the Winter Park Disabled Ski Team, I would be able to train with many of the racers and coaches of the U.S. Disabled Ski Team and even go to most of the races.

With this kind of practice, I would graduate high school one step ahead of the other skiers who want to make the U.S. Disabled Ski team in time for the 2006 Paralympics (the Olympics of disabled sports, held a few days after the regular Games in the same place).

To be able to do this next year (yes, my parents reluctantly agreed), I must raise $15,000. This goes toward living expenses, coaching fees, skiing equipment, race fees and plane tickets.

Unfortunately, I can't look for a corporate sponsor until I have a good racing record. My money must come from people, people who believe in me and where I'm going.

But my job as a racer is not to worry about money. I like to worry about holding an edge to the end of the turn and throwing my weight down the hill and finding the fastest line through the gates. I like to practice racing in my mind so many times that I feel I can reach out and touch the U.S. Disabled Ski Team sticker on the back of my car.

I want to put that sticker on my car when I've earned it.

I want to stand on the podium with a gold medal and thank all the people who believed in me.

I want to write a book that will inspire millions.

I want your kid to see my picture in the sports section, and I want you to tell him how I got there.

gym class determination

Originally published in *The Newsstreak*

Do you believe in destiny? I do. Not the fatalistic kind that gets you off the hook for not trying, but the kind of far off destiny that moves according to our habits and actions. Destiny is what a little boy on a balance beam sees in front of him. As he dips his toes beside the beam, his head bobs and destiny shifts for a few seconds. Sometimes, the boy does a cartwheel and destiny flips over. Every once in a while he falls from the beam and his destiny becomes a rubberized mat staring him in the face.

Time passes and the day of the big gymnastics meet arrives, but the boy can no longer walk on the balance beam. Instead, he hops over to the uneven bars and performs five pull-ups. His left leg, securely fastened in a gray brace, just dangles beneath him.

It was four years after that meet before I again had to do pull-ups. The new spectators were students in my freshman gym class. I did twenty. It's easy for me now because a leg is eighteen percent of your body weight. On the way back to my locker after that gym class, I bragged to myself that if I had really wanted it, I could've done twenty-five. I imagined something more inside of me just waiting to jump out if I could find a strong enough purpose. Where, I wondered, could I find such a purpose?

The search took me back to the days when I was in the hospital being doused with never ending doses of chemotherapy. Whenever the nurses took my temperature, they noticed I was exactly one degree colder than the average person; I always measured 97.6 degrees. In my body, 98.6 was a fever. This means winter affects me differently. I feel the cold like anyone else; it's just that I happen to thrive on it. I could live off a simple diet of water and chilly mornings.

Fortunately, there is not a colder moment than the few seconds before a ski race.

"Racer ready in ten, nine, eight, seven..." Like destiny, the course is always set for me, and the finish line drawn in the distance. I could stand still, and destiny would just sit there and wait for me to die. Or I could attack the mountain, bashing the gates with pull-up ready shoulders and sliding on a ski no wider than a balance beam.

Sometimes I think ski racing is my destiny and in a way, maybe it is. I believe life is a combination of seeing the path and choosing to walk on it. It's as if God wrote a beautiful script for my life, wrapped it up and gave it to me when I was born. It's up to me to rip it open and run with it.

No, destiny still moves when I move. It still dips when I dip and climbs when I climb, oscillating like the pull-ups for which I have finally found a purpose: I want stronger arms to bash slalom gates. I want a bigger chest to wear an Olympic medal. The other day I did twenty-six pull-ups.

gaining strength from success, failure

Originally published in *The Richmond Times-Dispatch*

Whenever I look at the poster of him on my wall, I hope someday I can ski like Greg Mannino, one of the best one-legged skiers in the world.

I finally got to meet him at the Columbia Crest Cup last month. Held in Winter Park, Colorado, it is the largest national qualifying race for U.S. Disabled Nationals, which are going on now. The Winter Park competition, a four-day event, draws disabled skiers from around the world – including me.

My first race was even better than I had hoped. I skied well and won the Juniors class (Note: The juniors class was, like, three people). After the awards ceremony, I introduced myself to Mannino. He's a big, lighthearted kind of guy with bleached-blond hair and a goatee.

"I haven't seen you ski yet," he said. "I will have to watch for you tomorrow."

I couldn't believe it! Greg Mannino, the guy on my wall, was going to watch for me! I decided my skiing would be great from then on, even better that the first day. The next morning, I burst out of the gate hungry for another victory. I tore through the course and tucked the last few gates. After crossing finish line, I checked the scoreboard. I'll never forget that moment: the thrill of victory mixed with surging adrenaline. What a great feeling! I had won Juniors two days in a row, and I hoped Greg would congratulate me.

I looked around. He was standing far off, joking with his friends. Obviously, he hadn't watched the race. My heart sank.

The third day was Giant Slalom, my worst event. You have to race twice on a curvy, icy course. Learning to ski in Virginia should have gotten me used to ice. It hadn't. I slid on every turn. I carried very little speed. After the first run, my time was far behind the other racers'.

I wanted to go up and erase my time so no one would see it. But there it was, plastered on the scoreboard. I was so far behind that even a near perfect second run wouldn't bring me into the lead. I was going to lose. Worst of all, my loss would stand out because I had won the first two races.

So I thought of an escape plan. Rather than face a slow time and a poor finish, I could purposely fall on my second run and get a DNF (did not finish). That way, no one would notice my time and I could pretend I had just skied too aggressively. Then I thought about it. Why risk getting hurt? I could just miss a gate or "accidentally" ski off the course. My record would be clean. Two races finished, two races won. I wouldn't accept defeat, I would just avoid it.

And for some reason, I wanted to avoid people as well.

I slipped into the competition center locker room and grabbed a Clif Bar and a book from my backpack. After wandering around a little, I found my way into the basement.

I sat down in the corner, took a bite out of my Chocolate Almond Fudge bar and picked up my book *Think and Grow Rich* by Napoleon Hill. The bookmark was in a chapter about decision.

I had already made my decision about the race, so I checked the next chapter. It was about persistence. I felt a twinge of guilt as I started to read.

"Lack of persistence is a weakness common to the majority of men."

I thought about this for a moment. I didn't want to be weak, and I certainly wasn't going to be common.

That was all it took. I would still lose the race, but I wasn't going to hang around with the "majority of men."

"Racer 57 in the gate," called the announcer.

That's me.

I will persist, I told myself at the starting gate. I will finish even if I'm in last place.

"Ten seconds."

I took a few quick deep breaths. Focus. Focus. I glanced down the course. Then, out of the corner of my eye, I saw him. Greg Mannino was standing near the gate, waiting for me to start. There were no buddies with him. Just Greg, watching me race.

"Racer ready in five, four, three, two…"

I burst out of the gate.

finding success on Mondays

Originally published in *The Richmond Times Dispatch*

The next time you need to practice your communication skills, try explaining why adults hate Mondays to a group of ten and eleven-year-olds.

"People always say how much they hate Mondays, and it's terrible, because one-seventh of your life is spent on Monday," said my friend Nick to Barbara Conley's fifth-grade class at Thelma Crenshaw Elementary School in Chesterfield County.

Thirty confused faces stared back at Nick. Scrambling for words I tried to help explain.

"When you get a little older, even by the time you are in high school, people will start to hate Mondays and feel sad, just because it's Monday. Some grown-ups especially do this because they don't want to go back to their jobs," I said.

They seemed even more confused.

"See, a lot of adults work at jobs they don't like," I said.

As if on cue, they shook their heads in amazement.

"Why would anyone do that?" a kid asked.

Nick and I, along with our friend Christian, were speechless. We tried to explain that, as sixteen-year-olds, it doesn't make a lot of sense to us, either, but it's true. A lot of people hate their jobs, and a lot of people hate Mondays.

On the other hand, we weren't there to complain about society. Actually, we went to Crenshaw because we believe there is hope for people to change.

a leg up

During our talks, the three of us gave the students a steady, hour-long stream of motivational clichés. Interestingly enough, none of the students seemed surprised that they had greatness within them or that they should create goals in their lives. This information apparently was common fifth-grade sense.

Then I noticed the classroom walls. Positive posters were plastered all over, including one with a giant highway that said: "The road to success – do your best."

I thought back to when I was their age. I saw posters like that all the time and believed them. The only problem was, I didn't really care. Success meant nothing to an average 11-year old like me. I mean, who wants "success" when you can play soccer or ride your bike with your friends?

Now I'm sixteen, and seeing a poster with the word "success" triggers all kinds of associations from my countless self-help books and motivational tapes. Now that I'm sixteen, I actually take the clichés seriously. Now I see that poster and want to do my best. I want success.

But now that I'm sixteen, I've also stubbed my toe a few times. I've seen problems bigger than my friend forgetting his lunch, and I've had failures worse than losing my homework. My challenges may even have been above normal: I've had cancer take away my leg and almost my Mom. But I keep believing the clichés and trying to instill them in others.

When we went to Crenshaw, Mrs. Conley joked that we must be crazy to give up a day of spring break to drive two hours to Chesterfield to talk with them. Actually, I think we are on track with what we want to do with our school assembly talks.

Don't ask me why I still believe in clichés, because I don't know. I just know that despite the challenges I've faced, I still see the road in front of me, and I want to travel it at top speed. I'm not interested in traveling on "reality" or some other dead-end road frequented by the kind of people who hate Mondays.

There are a lot of things I want, but there's one thing I'm really afraid of: getting comfortable. I'm scared of becoming satisfied. I'm scared that I will get tired of growing and will choose the easy road on Monday morning.

This reminds me of another cliché: Focus on what you want, not what you're afraid of.

And I do know what I want.

I want the energy, laughter and exuberance of the twenty-four fifth-graders in Mrs. Conley's class, and I want the drive of an adult ready to make it big in the world. I want all this, and I want it all the time, but especially on Monday mornings.

inspired to motivate

Originally published in *The Richmond Times Dispatch*

Motivational speakers are supposed to inspire you. They're supposed to make you laugh and, maybe, make you cry. But when Milton Creagh spoke at my high school two years ago, he made me jealous. It wasn't that I didn't like his speech. I loved it. The problem I had was really with me and a dream I had given up on. Back then, it seemed impossible. First of all, I doubted I had what it took to be a motivational speaker. Second, I was too young. Third, if I told people I wanted to speak professionally, they probably would laugh at me, and I hate criticism. Fourth, audiences might not like me. I hate rejection.

As I agonized over these fears, Creagh just kept on speaking, unaware of the conflict inside a 14-year old in the audience. I remember being amazed by his career. One of the premier high school speakers in the country, he has spoken to millions of teens in the past decade. And there I was, torn between my dream of being a speaker and the fear of what that could mean.

While I was wrestling with my decision, Creagh declared that a leader "has to have guts." Something snapped. I realized why I was there, in that seat, in that school. I realized why I had lost my leg to cancer and why I was still alive. God had given me a message, but I had only one life in which to spread it, and only one way to do it. I grabbed a pen and scribbled "a leader has guts" on my arm.

I walked away from that talk a different person. No longer was I another high school student. No longer was I another cancer survivor. I was a motivational speaker.

Many people did laugh—literally—when I told them I wanted to speak. They seamed to think it was impossible. Maybe it was, but I had a fire burning inside, and I wanted to speak to anyone who would listen.

My talks went well, and I became a decent speaker. But I knew I was just decent, not great, because great speakers got paid. I didn't. I knew that an outstanding speaker has potential clients asking, "What's your fee?" I needed to improve, and the only way to do so was to practice. So I kept looking for more opportunities.

Just last month, I called the director of a youth leadership camp and tried to persuade him to let me speak for free. Even though the conference began in three days, he said he would try. When he didn't call back, I just showed up at the camp. I wandered around for two hours looking for him. When I finally found him, the director told me that the schedule was full, but he would arrange for me to speak to the teachers who were there. Then I spoke for my allotted 10 minutes about overcoming obstacles.

As I concluded, a woman raised her hand and asked whether I could speak at her school. "Of course," I said. Then another hand went up in the back of the room. "Yeah?" I said, motioning to the raised arm.

"How much do you charge?" asked the teacher.

I was speechless. I tried to make up a number, but no words came out of my mouth. This was the question I had been waiting to hear since Creagh spoke at my school two years before. Literally at that same instant, all eyes turned to the door as the next speaker entered the room. In walked none other than the big man himself, Milton Creagh. As he approached the podium, I told him what happened when he spoke at my school.

"If it wasn't for this guy, I wouldn't be speaking to you today!" I told the audience. They applauded.

Moments later, Creagh gave me his assistant's phone number.

"I'm going to have to retire soon," he said, referring to his commitment to be host of a talk show. "Call me."

"I will," I said. "I definitely will."

trio discovers the power of a dream

Originally published in *The Richmond Times Dispatch*

I sat down on the edge of the stage and took a deep breath. The auditorium was completely empty except for the few of us drifting around the stage.

I'd always assumed that I'd have a feeling of accomplishment after our first assembly. I had recruited a team of speakers from my high school, found a corporate sponsor and then booked a few dates at area middle schools. But instead of accomplishment, I felt only the effects of a late-night rehearsal and five hours of sleep.

This was the day Nick Mestre, Christian Jackson and I presented our first motivational program for middle schools at Pence Middle School in Dayton, Virginia.

We had just finished assemblies with the seventh and then, eighth graders. It had been our dream that these would be the first of many assemblies. But sitting there on the stage, I just remembered all the little things that went wrong that morning:

- Our disastrous attempt to hold a dance contest
- We tried to show some videos we had produced, but a cable in the video projector short-circuited and "error" messages appeared periodically
- Christian's wireless microphone went out during his speech

At least Nick's talk about self-esteem had seemed to connect with the kids. And my speech at the end about my battle with cancer seemed to work. I explained how to create powerful goals by deciding what you want, writing it down and taking immediate action. We finished by singing and dancing to our 'N Sync parody of "It's Gonna Be Me." (We changed the words to "It's Gonna Be Dreams.")

In our assemblies, we challenged the nearly three-hundred students to come forward at the end and commit their goals to paper. We called it the "Jones Challenge" after our sponsor, Jones Soda, and we had forms ready to fill out. We had hoped for 50 responses, but when we dismissed, virtually all of the students came forward to write down a goal and an action step to accomplish that day.

A very large crowd of eager goal setters seemed like a nice problem to have, but several teachers were angry with the chaos and began herding students back to class. We were supposed to do three assemblies, but the principal canceled our third program because of scheduling problems.

So there we were in the empty auditorium, the three of us contemplating our disastrous first attempt at becoming motivational speakers. Lost in my thoughts, I didn't even see a girl walk down the aisle, hand Nick a folded sheet of notebook paper, and leave. Seconds later, he elbowed me.

"Read this," he said.

I took the letter addressed "Hey Guys," and my eyes began to read: "My real mother got hooked on crack cocaine and crank. She went to rehab, but she was kicked out of it. She backslid. My younger brother is a drug baby."

Her note went on to tell about her uncle who used to live with her "family." He was an alcoholic who abused his girlfriend and destroyed the house.

"Everything in my life was so messed up. I couldn't wait to either leave or end up in such a depression I couldn't eat," the letter continued.

"When you guys came along and started talking about morals and goals, I decided I want to set some, too.

"I want to be a tattoo artist and have lots of business. I love you guys."

It was signed with an email address and simple instructions to read her letter to people so "they know it is not too late for them."

I handed the letter to Christian.

Then, motioning toward the stack of goal sheets completed by hundreds of kids that morning, I spoke the only words that came to mind: "This is as good as it gets."

be your own beat master and lead

Originally published in *The Richmond Times Dispatch*

In case you were wondering, starting a band a week after purchasing your very first drum set is a bad idea. I know because I did it. At the time, I didn't even know the names of the different drums, much less how to play them. But Jonathan and I were convinced that record companies were scouring the country for new musical talent of the middle school variety, and would probably sign us as soon as we wrote our first song. So we combined instruments and became a cliché: The teen rock band.

Normally, the drummer's job is to keep the rhythm of the song. In my case, I had absolutely no ability to stay on time.

"Don't worry if you get offbeat," Jonathan said at our first practice. "I can probably just change the guitar tempo to match your new beat."

Grateful for this newfound freedom, I banged on random cymbals and drums whenever it seemed appropriate.

A few months later, we recruited Patrick, a bass player. Not only was he a fantastic bass player, he also played the drums. And, unlike me, he was very good.

This made my new job even scarier. Patrick would suggest a new, complicated beat.

"Just hit that drum and that symbol and then this drum..."

I would agree and then I would change the subject of conversation until he and Jonathan forgot the idea, allowing me to return to the "basic rock beat." The truth was, anything more complicated scared me. I didn't want to risk messing up. I didn't want Jonathan and Patrick to look at me funny when I got offbeat. I just wanted to fit in with the music.

I'll never forget our debut performance at our church's talent night. We were attempting to be a Christian band so we thought it was a good match. It would have been better had I known how to play the drums and control my stage fright. As it was, I looked out in that auditorium filled with 300 expectant faces and could barely remember my "basic rock beat." So paralyzing was my fear of making a mistake that I hit the drums with the amount of force I normally reserve for petting kittens.

I thought everything would be OK when it was over, but I was wrong. If we could've sold a CD for every time someone told us, "Cool song, but I couldn't hear the drums," we would've gone multi-platinum that very night.

I kept all these things inside until Matt came to "mess around" with us at practice. I quickly noticed he was one of those guys who's so musically talented you don't know whether to love him or hate him. He could play every instrument better than we could.

After we played a song for him, he made a statement that exposed all that I'd worked so hard to hide.

"Josh, you're not supposed to play along with the music," he said. "You're supposed to set the beat. You're the leader of the band."

This idea had never really occurred to me. I learned how to play the drums by playing along with CD's so it seemed natural to play along with what I was hearing. Add to that my debilitating fear of making a mistake and standing out and I had a recipe for failure in drumming.

Or in life.

Fast forward five years to the present and come with me to a middle school auditorium in Alexandria. As the students file into the room for a motivational assembly program, they see a teen-age guy playing drums up front. He's trying to get kids to freestyle rap.

The guy on the drums isn't the best musician, but no one seems to care. He keeps a good hip-hop beat and the kids love it. Some are dancing. Some are clapping. Some are even rapping.

The guy on the drums no longer worries about being off or making a mistake. That's not important anymore. He's setting his own beat.

parents spout illogical wisdom
Originally published in *The Newsstreak*

From the time we were born, our mothers have been repeating factually unsound admonishments. I am writing this column to expose them once and for all.

"Don't cross your eyes or they'll get stuck that way."
I tried this. It didn't work.

"Don't do that – you'll poke your eye out!"
It is impossible to poke your eye out. Ask any doctor. You can you can poke it *in*, sure, but not *out*. You have to gorge it out.

"A penny saved is a penny earned."
Classic logical fallacy known as "If A, then B." Just because the penny was saved does not mean that it was also earned. I could easily steal a penny from my younger brother and save it. Does this mean I earned it? Of course not! I prefer this slogan: "A penny saved – is not very much."

Spelling
When I was little, we still had to figure out how to spell words without the help of a spell checker on the computer. Whenever I wanted to know how to spell a word, I would call out the word to my Mom from my bedroom.
"How do you spell it?" I would yell.

"Look it up in the dictionary!" was invariably her response.

"HOW CAN I LOOK IT UP IF I DON'T KNOW HOW TO SPELL IT?"

Arguing

This illogic is all too common with parents. For example, a parent might angrily yell, "Look at me when I'm talking to you!" And a moment later say, "Don't look at me that way!"

"Finish your food because children in China are starving."

How does the amount of food I eat have one iota of effect on starving children in China? I think it is just the opposite. If I don't finish my food, perhaps it would fall out of the garbage truck, and float across the ocean to China! If I eat all my food, on the other hand, there is absolutely no chance of this happening.

America Online doesn't know Chinese

Originally published in *The Newsstreak*

Nowadays, my younger siblings laugh at stories about when I had to record my time on America Online. Only a select few internet users can remember back in the day when you couldn't exceed the 40-hour-a-month maximum. I've met fellow old timers who soared past their maximum hours, driving their AOL bill past $500.

Back in the day, a new AOL member got their first 30 hours online for free. A few weeks ago, I got an AOL CD in the mail that declared "FIRST 700 HOURS FREE!" (In small letters at the bottom, the package said that these 700 must be used in a month.)

I felt cheated. Not because I only got 30 free hours when I joined, but because AOL was obviously trying to steal several hours from new members who join in February.

Let me explain. At its normal 28 days, February has a total of only 672 hours. Even on a leap year, February has only 696 hours. Outraged, I called AOL's customer support line (800-827-6364) to clear up this misunderstanding. What follows is the transcript of our conversation on 10/27/00 at 11:16 a.m. (Note that I talked very slow as if I was always confused):

AOL: Hi this is Tamra, how can I help you?

Me: Yes, I got a disc in the mail that tells me I have 700 free hours on AOL, but I am going to get a computer and start using AOL in February. Since February only has 672 hours, I was wondering if there was any way I could use up the other 30 hours. Maybe I could use two computers at once?

Tamra: No, the hours are take it or leave it.

Me: But I want to get my money's worth. How could I use the full 700 hours?

Tamra: Actually, you get a full month. Like if you signed on February 2nd, you would have till March 2nd.

Me: Oooh. How many days is that?

Tamra: You get 30 days.

Me: So I have a full 720 hours to use up my time.

Tamra: Yes.

Me: I have another problem though. I like to sleep at night and during that time I don't think I could be online. Is there anyway I could hook up with someone, perhaps in China, who could use my account at night? That way I could make sure I use up the full 700 hours.

Tamra: You can use your account however you want.

Me: What happens if we run out of the 700 hours, but there are still 20 hours left in the month?

Tamra: Actually, we don't keep track of the hours. You get unlimited time for a month.

Me: What?! Isn't that false advertising?

(Try as I might, I couldn't make Tamra mad. However I often heard muffled laughter).

Tamra: Well, if you call us, then we tell you.

Me: But what if I didn't call?

Tamra: The disc can tell you when you start using it.

Me: OK, thank you. You have been very helpful. Do you happen to know anyone in China who would want to share an AOL account?

Tamra: No, sorry, I don't.

Me: You don't speak Chinese, do you?

Tamra: [Click]

awareness strengthens our democracy
Originally published in the *The Newsstreak*

Many people claim that America has a strong economy, army and government. They say that the United States is a shining light on a hill in a dark, communist world. These things are all notable, but they are truly insignificant when we consider the most fundamental element of a society: Awareness.

Specifically, we thrive because of our ability to designate specific periods of time for the promotion of particular issues and concepts. For example, where would we be without National Neurofibromatosis Awareness Month in May? Without this awareness of disease, how could we learn that the most common form of Neurofibromatosis is Recklinghausen?

Indeed, our country's fully aware calendar is the underlying reason for a thriving economy. Let's consider the full year starting with January. Everything kicks off in January, with National Glaucoma Awareness Month. And how could anyone keep their New Year's resolution if January wasn't also Rotary Awareness Month?

It's really unfortunate that February is so short. If it were a few days longer, I could squeeze in a few more parties to celebrate Humpback Whales Awareness Month. (Humpback Whales love leap year).

March is also a very important month. Parenting Awareness Month always reminds me to enjoy my days as a youth as much as possible. March also happens to be Women's Awareness Month. If you ask me, men are always aware of women the other eleven months of the year anyway. (Maybe I'm

a leg up

just bitter because there's no Men's Awareness Month). Of course, music fans across the country celebrate March as Bass Player's Awareness Month.

Who could forget that April is Math Awareness Month? Millions of students get up in the morning everyday simply because they know April is coming.

Besides Neurofibromatosis, May is the month to be aware of "Older Americans." You might think that Older Americans Awareness Month would incite annual riots of envy in foreign nursing homes everywhere, but remember, other countries generally don't value awareness like we do in the United States. (There is one exception to this rule: Strokes. Canada celebrates Stroke Awareness Month for a full month in June, and Britain celebrates it all of May, but the United States gives strokes just one lousy week in September).

Moving on to June, which is National Helen Keller Deaf-Blind Awareness Week. If anyone knows about that one—and I'm not sure anyone does—I suspect they probably just use it as an excuse to make Helen Keller jokes.

July and August don't have any celebrations that a true American wouldn't already be aware of. For example, August is Skin Cancer Awareness Month. The fact is, it doesn't take a mega-aware person to notice skin on their own body. If McCain can do it, so can you.

Most people don't know that September 18-22 is Prostate Cancer Awareness Week. These all important seven days lose attention to our country's true love: Breast Cancer Awareness Month in October. Don't get me wrong – mammograms are great and everything, but we shouldn't overlook the men of our society.

In my research, I could not find any awareness celebrations in December. This is probably because we spend most of our time trying to be aware of any reference to "Christmas" on government property during December. However, I think that trashing Nativity Scenes isn't enough for December. Perhaps December should be a generic "Awareness Month" to help us all be more cognizant of our awareness. I would want nothing more for my Holiday Season than to gather around the tree and recount memories from great celebrations like Professional Secretaries Week in April and Visit Your Relatives Day on May 18th. If our country could make this kind of commitment to awareness, I believe it would be a big step forward for democracy.

guide to surviving hallway rudeness

Originally published in *The Newsstreak*

I often wonder. Do they not see me, or is the floor really that interesting? I mean, I played hop-scotch when I was five, but generally, high schoolers have gotten over their fascination with floor design. It's just a bunch of squares, people!

I don't think I'll ever understand rudeness. These people stare at the floor and mindlessly walk through the hall crowds. They run into you, and keep walking. If you don't move to the side, they will just keep walking and push you with them.

This can be a bad situation when the halls are very crowded. I believe I have developed some solutions. If you have no space to the left or right, and someone is plowing you along, first try the verbal technique. Yell something like, "I love school!" I guarantee the entire school will stop and look at you. A variation of this is yelling, "My, how I love school lunches!" Several students around the country have been beat up using this technique.

When the above verbal techniques fail, try an idea that has since been adapted for fire safety. It's called stop, drop, and roll. When you notice a head pounding into your stomach, try stop, drop, and roll. First stop. Don't try to walk forward; it will just make things worse. Drop to the floor. Next is the tricky part: You must roll under the person's legs, continue rolling and stand up all in on motion. This action seems to turn heads of other students, so be sure to have a pen out to take phone numbers.

Still, I can't understand why these people just don't look up. Unless your neck is broken (in which case you shouldn't be bumping into people anyway), there is no excuse for not being able to lift one's head. I mean, can't they just lift their head high enough to look at you? Rude hallway people remind me of blind drivers. (Yes, they exist. I know one of them).

Another problem with rudeness: People who don't wear deodorant. Please. Wear. Deodorant. Especially if you are going to bump into people. It should be a school rule that if you are going to run into people in the hallway, you must wear deodorant, you must use breath mints, and you must not have eaten a cafeteria lunch within the past two hours.

how to anger fast food employees
Originally published in *The Newsstreak,*

This summer, a few friends and I decided to solve a problem that uncreative people have wrestled with for centuries. What do you do for fun as a teenager in a small town?

We decided to harass fast food drive thru employees.

On our first day, Kent Barnes and Robert Gu came over to my house with a video camera. They insisted that I drive, despite that it was my first week driving after my sixteenth birthday ("I don't have any gas," claimed Kent). So we all piled into my little Toyota, and drove to Burger King.

We started with an easy one, number ten on the list. The camera running in the passenger seat, the conversation went like this:

"Hi, welcome to Burger King, can I take your order?"

"Yes, I'll have a small chocolate Coke and a large Jr. fry, hold the pickles."

Long pause.

"That's a small chocolate shake, a Coke, and Jr. Whopper with out the pickles?"

"No, the chocolate is in the Coke, and hold the pickles on the fries."

Another pause.

"Uh, just drive around for your total."

(We didn't).

Next I drove to Hardees. Kent went to hide behind a telephone poll with the video camera, and Robert got in the trunk.

I ordered, and pulled around to pick up my double cheeseburger. At this point, Robert started banging on the trunk and screaming.

"HELP! SOMEONE LET ME OUT OF HERE! PLEASE!"

This went on while I paid and received my food. Finally, the guy at the window leaned out a little and pointed toward my trunk.

"What is-"

I cut him off with a cheerful, "Thank you!"

On this cue, Robert popped the trunk open. He made a mad dash across the parking lot, screaming about freedom like a warrior in Braveheart.

In one of our boldest moves, we went to a Wendy's wearing nothing but strategically placed seatbelts. Unfortunately, it turned out that the girl at the drive-thru window was my next door neighbor. (Note: You may think I am making this up. But I can assure you that it was true, and things were subsequently very awkward whenever we ran into each other at the mailbox).

Since you can't ever understand those drive thru speakers, we decided to turn the tables and distort our own voices. At Taco Bell, for example, Kent sucked some helium and made his order. At McDonald's, I spoke in totally nonsensical phrases and noises. Another time, I used the classic technique to get the employee to turn up the earphones by whispering your order several times. Then I YELLED the order.

Let me close by sharing the best and worst responses we got from an employee.

Best: A girl at Arby's gave me a 10% discount for telling her a joke.

Worst: At McDonald's. Before he could greet me, I leaned out the window and shouted enthusiastically, "Hi, welcome to McDonald's, can I take your order please?"

As planned, we all burst out into hysterical laughter in the car.

"Hello," I repeated. "Can I take your order?"

Finally came a deeply irritated voice.

"Can I HELP you?"

"Yes, I'd like a small Coke please."

"No."

"No small Cokes?"

"No."

Disclaimer: Do not try this at home. Fast food drive thru employees work very hard and should not have to put up with people like my friends and me. I apologize to all fast food people who were harmed during the creation of this column.

Want to watch Josh's original "Fast Food Drive Thru Pranks" video? *See page 102 for details.*

states of being

Originally published in *The Newsstreak*

I think the only time I feel comfortable saying I'm "bad" is in Spanish class. When we are surveyed at the start of first period, we can all choose if we are "bien" or "mal." Sometimes I pick mal, just because I get tired of always saying I am "good" in my everyday English conversations.

Let's be honest: We are all tired of small talk. In fact, we are so tired of it that we are getting it confused. How many times have you had this conversation?

You: "How are you?"

Zombie: "Not much, dude!"

You: "No, *how* are you?"

Zombie: "Fine, what's up with you?"

You: "Good, what's going on with you?"

Zombie: "Errr...Nothing."

I finally got to hear some new small talk last spring when I met motivational speaker Zig Ziglar. He's always been proud of his enthusiasm and positive thinking, and even at age seventy-two he remains in an abnormal state of being. I will never forget when I asked, "How are you doing, Mr. Ziglar?" and he declared that he was "better than good." What can you say to that?

This kind of abnormal state of being caused me to want to feel better myself. So this year I decided to be awesome. "I'm awesome, how about you?" was how I started conversations for the first month of school. But I found that feeling good made other people feel guilty for having such a lame adjective as "well."

Eventually, I got tired of this, so I assembled a list of states of being that no one would ever expect. I went to school prepared to floor any zombies interested in small talk. The first opportunity came in the men's room before first period.

My friend, Chris, was using a urinal to my right.

"How are you?" said unsuspecting Chris, following etiquette by staring at the wall.

"Ballistic, how are you?" I said smiling.

Chris looked around nervously.

All day, I kept throwing new words out there. I was "impassioned," "phenomenal," or "satiated with joy."

Yes, I am smashing spectacular. What's up with you?

faith and dreams

Originally published in *The Newsstreak*

Almost a year later, I still remember that chart. It had a block for every year from 2001 until 2006, the year I hope to ski in the Paralympics.

"See, look," I said to my skeptical parents. "If I wait to train until after high school, that's only three seasons before 2006. I need to start training my senior year." I filled in the 2001-2002 ski season with my pen.

"There are a lot of other people who want a medal. To win, I have to train more than them," I said.

My parents silently mulled over my competitive strategy.

"We'll think and pray about it," my Dad finally said. "There are a lot of big things that need to happen before you can go, and if God wants you to go, they will work out."

I hated the inconclusiveness of his answer, but I knew he was right. There was money to be raised (an intimidating $15,000), there was the high school diploma issue, and even if those problems were solved, where would I live?

On the other hand, the Bible says God gives us the desires of our heart. You could say this means God gives you everything you want, but I don't really think that's accurate. I think it means that the desires, the dreams we have come from God. And if that's true, then skiing seemed to be something God wanted for me. And I had faith that if God was on my side, He could definitely take care of the details along the way.

My parents, on the other hand, were not quite so convinced. And being parents, they were very worried...about everything. For example, my Mom was worried about whether or not I would have a church to attend. So she somehow acquired the e-mail address of a family who lived in a town near the ski resort and wrote them about my situation. A few e-mails later, the family decided out of the blue that they wanted me to stay with them, if I was interested. They were offering free lodging and they had a teenage son who was my own age, so I gratefully accepted the invitation.

Harrisonburg High School Principal Irene Reynolds and Superintendent Dr. Donald Ford were very helpful in making arrangements for my second semester. Since HHS began offering classes over the Internet for the first time this year, getting all my credits scheduled turned out to be pretty easy. Then, a manager at the Ski Chalet in Richmond called a representative from Rossignol and convinced him to give me skis. A deal like this is amazing, because it normally takes racers several seasons before they are getting any free equipment, and here I was in my second season, racing on top of the line equipment that was given to me free.

Between the free skies and staying with the family, the tab on my season had come down to only $10,000. Now, I just need to find a way to raise it. One day I received a call out of nowhere from a total stranger named Linda Tobin.

"Listen, Josh," she said. "I heard you need to raise money for skiing."

"Yeah, I do."

"Well, I used to do fund-raising professionally, and I want to help you."

This conversation turned into an amazing direct mail fund-raising drive over the summer. Although I helped design the materials and write the letters, Linda Tobin developed the address list and stuffed every single envelope. By November, I had raised the $10,000 and then some.

Now you might not believe in God, and that's your choice, but I personally see no other explanation for the way my ski racing dreams have become a reality so quickly. I wouldn't have said this a year ago, but if you really have faith in a dream, and if God's behind what you're doing, I believe you become like a magnet, attracting everything you need to achieve the goal.

Like I said, if you had told me that a year ago, I would've thought you were a bit crazy, or at least overly idealistic. Now I'm convinced that the faith of a mustard seed can move mountains, or, in my case, move you to the mountains.

renewed hunger helps refocus

Originally published in *The Richmond Times Dispatch*

You know those anti-depressant commercials? The ones where they say sleeplessness is a symptom of depression? Well, what do you call it if you can't sleep because you're too happy?

After I moved to Colorado in mid-January, I was so excited about skiing that I just couldn't fall asleep at night.

My energy and spirits had never been higher. I was working out twice a day, plus training for ski racing in the morning and afternoon. I should've been tired at night, but there I was, staring at the ceiling above my bed.

I also had this problem with being happy. When you ski poorly, you want to get upset so you will have the motivation to change – and do better – on the next run. But I just couldn't do it. Even after a bad day of skiing, I remained incessantly happy.

Like I said, it wasn't depression.

I was on top of the world. I felt like Romeo after meeting Juliet. Like a blind man after seeing the world for the first time. Nothing could stop me. Not even lack of sleep or a bad run.

Everyday I was totally focused on my goals: the U.S. Disabled Ski Team and the Paralympics in 2006. My focus on these goals was like the sun through a magnifying glass. I felt ready to melt the snow on any ski course on the mountain.

But gradually, my euphoria began to fade and something else took its place. And like with many disorders, I didn't recognize the symptoms until it was almost too late. It started with sleeping. That is, I was falling asleep just fine and I was no longer happy when I heard the alarm in the morning. And then, at practice, I sometimes wanted to be somewhere else. Somewhere warm. I used to be hungry for cold, but suddenly, I was putting on bunches of layers before I went on the snow.

And so I sat back as complacency crept up on my dream. Then, one day at practice, it all came crashing down. I couldn't get psyched up to go down the hill. I couldn't seem to finish the course. Everything felt terribly wrong.

I had the next day off, and it was the kind of day you'd expect at 10,000 feet: cold and windy with a snowstorm so thick I couldn't see the neighbor's house.

A nice day for a run.

I donned my shorts (I always run in shorts), my sunglasses (to block the snow from my eyes) and went out into the storm. As I skipped along through the snow, I left the telltale tracks of someone running with two crutches and one leg.

I thought about my first few weeks in Colorado. I thought about fund-raising for this trip over the summer and the daily trips to the gym before school. And then I wondered why, after I'd come so far, was I losing sight of my future?

In an icy instant, as a freezing burst of snow whipped through my shorts and sweatshirt, the answer seemed to jump out of the wind. I had lost my hunger!

It had been my hunger to compete that had brought me to ski racing a year before. It was my hunger to be the best that had brought me to Colorado for the season. And now, though I was neither the best nor particularly competitive, I had let a little taste of my dream be enough to satisfy my cravings.

This, I told myself, was sick. I have only one life to live and I refuse to live in such a way that I can be satisfied by only a small bite of what is truly possible. No, I want to be insatiable when it comes to fulfilling my dreams!

Every day when I go out to train, I must be hungry for progress, for improvement. The moment I am satisfied with my skiing is the moment I begin to regress and grow disinterested.

Whenever I go out for a race, I must be hungry for victory, not just hungry to cross the finish line because that hunger is not enough to help me win.

Victory, of course, is not yet mine, and often it seems too far off to even see it. But on days when I get discouraged, I just find an area where I can improve, and suddenly, that euphoria is back. Suddenly, I'm happy even when I fall.

small wins on road to meeting big goals

Originally published in *The Richmond Times Dispatch*

Before stripping down to my ski racing suit as I entered the starting gate, I had faint hopes that the suit was designed to keep the skier warm. It took just a few bursts of freezing wind for me to discern that this was not true.

Despite the incredibly icy and foggy conditions, my total lack of experience and the fact that I was the only racer there with one leg, I had high hopes for this race. I had planned to take the course by storm and win the whole thing. That was what I told myself as I tripped the starting wand and passed the first gate. About three turns into the course, I was flat on my back, my single ski somewhere above me on the hill. My second run wasn't much better. I went down five times, and each fall against the ice got a bit more painful and made me a little more angry. The snow was so granular that I cut my face on it—even though I had a face guard on my helmet. Some odd determination possessed me, however, and I kept getting back up until I crossed the finish line.

Not surprisingly, I got last place. My time was a whopping five times longer than the winning time, but this was still a victory – a symbol of strength and persistence I wanted to bring to my races. Even more important, I had gotten started on a dream of racing for the U.S. Disabled Ski Team in the 2006 Paralympics. Although my times didn't prove it, I had made progress by getting started, and progress is a form of victory in itself.

A year later, in January 2002, I returned to that same annual race in West Virginia. This time, I arrived with several competitions under my belt, even a few minor victories. But my victories had all been in races for disabled athletes. I wanted to beat some two-legged skiers this year to show them that I could hold my own even with one leg.

This year, the sun came out to soften the snow a bit. And, unlike last year's foggy view from the starting gate, I could see the finish line. I tripped the starting wand and entered the course feeling smooth, fast and aggressive. In the finish area, the announcer read my time: a quick 31 seconds, just two seconds behind most of the leaders and faster than many racers. I was elated.

My second run didn't feel as smooth, and I fell behind by a few more seconds. I was disappointed, but I obviously had made progress since last year, and, as I say, progress is victory. Unfortunately, personal victories often fail to translate into public victories, so I skipped the awards ceremony that afternoon. The next morning, while booting up for a second day of racing, one of my teammates turned to me.

"Hey, Josh, did you get your medal?"

"What?" I said.

"You got fifth place."

I smiled and thanked him. Six people were in my age category the previous day, so fifth place meant I had beaten just one guy. Not really a medal-deserving accomplishment, but fifth place represented something that was very important to me: I had beaten a racer who had two legs. I was disabled, but I was competitive on the able-bodied level.

Of course, first place would've been much better, but beating one guy meant progress from beating no one the year before. In the pursuit of a far-off victory like a Paralympic gold medal, I believe in finding smaller victories in the one thing I know I can get out of every day: progress.

I write this column from Winter Park, Colorado, where I have moved for three months to train for skiing full time. The thing that excites me most about being here is the opportunity to focus single-mindedly on a big goal and then celebrate the daily victories I made by improving.

I never did find out if anyone picked up my fifth-place medal. On the other hand, I don't care so much about the medal anymore, because now that I'm training daily, I have the opportunity to relive the victory of progress every single day.

dreams come at a price worth paying

Originally published in *The Richmond Times Dispatch*

Our plan was to skip the line by taking the handicapped entrances, thus beating some of the crowd in the race for a good seat. It was a simple decision, but it soon transformed our experience at the Paralympic Games downhill race.

Ralph and I, both one-legged skiers training for the 2006 Paralympics, just wanted to get as close a seat as possible. But when we saw the finish area just ahead of the handicapped entrance, we looked at each other and started walking in that direction. I could hardly believe they would allow spectators so close to the race, but no one said anything. Before I knew it, we were standing right beside the finish line.

"Sweet," I said.

Ralph nodded.

It wasn't long, however, before things didn't seem quite right. There were fences surrounding the area where we were, and I noticed uniformed Paralympic volunteers standing guard at the entrances. Beside us was a large tent from which people were emerging with food and drinks. And these were not just any people. They were the disabled athletes competing in the games.

"How are spectators allowed to be in the same area as the athletes?" I wondered. Then it hit me. Spectators aren't allowed in the same area as the athletes. I looked at Ralph, and in the same instant, we both realized where we were. I quickly pieced it together. The volunteers guarding the gates had assumed we were competitors because of our disabilities, so they let us in the athlete-only area. All we did was show up, walk in and suddenly we were among the top disabled skiers in the world.

It's funny. If you had asked me a year ago, I think that situation is how I would've described my goals in ski racing. I figured I could just show up at a race, ski through the finish line and suddenly I'd be among the top disabled skiers in the world.

But reality didn't quite match my fantasies. I did show up at the races, but I got stomped by the top athletes. And even though I've been training in Colorado this year, I haven't been doing much better in competition.

So many times I've wished I could just press a button and start winning races. But if such a button does exist, I have yet to find it.

Anyway, I wasn't thinking about these disappointments while we watched the race in Salt Lake. Instead, I was thinking about how great it would be to come onto that final pitch and hear 5,000 fans cheering you on at the finish.

I was thinking about what it would feel like to cross the finish line, look up at the scoreboard and see a "1st" beside my name. I was also thinking how fun it was to hang out in the finish area during the race. I loved the Coke machine in the hospitality tent that had the word "FREE" on the screen that normally displayed a price. You could just walk in, press any button and out popped the 20-oz beverage of your choice. While I admit being a sucker for anything that's free, I noticed something interesting. Many of the athletes would take a few sips and then leave the rest of the drink out on the table.

Why?

Because it was free. They didn't have to work for it or do anything to earn the soda. They just showed up at the tent, pressed the button and the drink popped out. That led me to a final question: If something as simple as a drink loses value when it's available at the press of a button, how much more meaningless would it be if I found a button that would grant me victory in ski racing?

So now, instead of looking for buttons labeled "free," you can find me on the slopes working hard and sacrificing to get into a finish area called "victory."

awaiting 2006

Originally published in *The Newsstreak*

Losing is for losers no matter what country you're in. Don't get me wrong, I had an awesome time being in Canada, but there's a fine line between getting motivated to make improvements in your skiing and getting discouraged about how many improvements need to be made. As for my first World Cup race, the results leaned towards discouraging.

After the race, I began to second guess myself. Maybe my body structure was not right for ski racing. Maybe I didn't have the personality it takes to win. Maybe I was in the wrong sport. Maybe my goals were impossible.

I mulled over all this during the seventeen hour drive from Kimberly, Canada to Salt Lake City, Utah where we were going to train in Park City and then watch some of the Paralympics.

On the night of the Paralympic opening ceremonies, the energy in the Olympic stadium was unbelievable. The arena was packed with some fifty-four thousand people, more than the number that attended opening ceremonies at the Olympics. The show was complete with fireworks, ice dancers, and performances by the likes of Stevie Wonder, Wynona and Donny Osmond.

Just like at the regular Olympics, the entrance of the athletes took forever as endless countries you've never heard of passed by. And just like at the regular Olympics, the place erupted when the U.S. Team entered the track. American flags waved everywhere, and the athletes pumped their fists and waved at the crowd.

I nudged one of my Winter Park teammates.

"That's us in four years," I said.

He nodded.

After the ceremonies had ended, while we waited for our coach to get the team van, the stadium totally cleared out. We were left alone with the volunteers and event crew members who were tearing down equipment.

Although I lacked credentials (the ID badge that allows you into restricted areas), I figured most people would assume a guy with one leg was one of the athletes. So, I decided to take a risk and walk onto the platforms in the middle of the arena.

Still feeling inspired from the opening ceremonies, I climbed out of the stands and walked down the runway that the athletes had circled during their entrance to the Paralympics.

In the ceremony, it seemed that every speaker and performer who stepped on the stage talked about one thing: Doing the impossible. I guess it doesn't sound like much more than a cliché, but the phrase struck a chord with a certain seventeen-year-old who was wondering whether his dreams were impossible.

Impossible? Wasn't that the essence of the Olympic spirit? Going after the impossible until it becomes possible?

Before I left the stadium, I decided to take one more stop. I walked up on the main stage, right to the middle, and just stood there. I imagined what it would feel like to be standing there with a medal around my neck, and with the stands totally full.

"Can I take your picture?"

The sudden question jolted me out of my victorious daydream.

"What?"

"Can I take a picture of you standing there?" the stranger repeated.

"I'm not competing in the games," I said hesitantly, figuring he'd only want to take a picture of a Paralympic athlete.

"That's OK," he said, kneeling down so the torch would be in the photo behind me.

"I will hopefully be there in 2006," I added.

"Well, tell you what," he said as he clicked the shudder a few times.

"If you make it in 2006, I will take your picture there, too."

I smiled.

"It's a deal," I said. "I'll be there."

showered with inspiration

originally published in *TeenSpeak*

I've heard that great minds think their best ideas in the shower. I am pleased to announce that I am now a part of this elite circle of creative thinkers. Last summer, as I was finishing up my morning shower, a crazy idea hit me: I wanted to put together a devotional book written by and for young people around the world. The title? *Forty Voices: Stories of Hope from Our Generation.* You are now reading the account of what happened (and what I learned) after I toweled off.

1. **You've got to bring enthusiasm to the table**. The first thing I did in my newfound cleanliness was to call two of my friends and ask them to join me as editors in the project. While I was dialing their numbers I recall having the feeling that my stomach was about to explode. Not from indigestion, mind you, but from sheer excitement. I really wanted to do this, and that excitement got the two of them interested, too.
2. **There's no "I" in team.** The more cynical among you will observe that there is in fact a "me" in team. This, however, is irrelevant. The three-man editing team of *Forty Voices* showed me just how powerful teamwork can be. Brian Hamilton, a high school buddy of mine and web designer, created a web page that we used to solicit entries. Brad Huddleston, being a radio disc jockey, got us radio time and pulled a few other nifty publicity stunts. And me? I've learned a good bit about publishing while working on an as-of-yet-unfinished autobiography, so I was in charge of the

logistics of publishing. The three of us were a match made in heaven. Literally.

3. **People are generally very irresponsible.** The more cynical among you are probably agreeing here. But it's true – getting people to follow through on their word and submit devotional stories for *Forty Voices* was a tough job. I can't tell you how many people told me, "I'll write something and email it to you tomorrow" and were never heard from again.

4. **Honesty is the best policy.** Our philosophy in writing a Christian book that would impart spiritual principles to the reader was to have our writers tell a story from their life that affected their relationship with God. We didn't want preaching, we wanted honesty. But that's hard because we all want to make ourselves out to be Perfect Christians. The truth is, no one is perfect, and it's only by admitting this that we can write about our lives in such a way that we connect with the reader.

5. **Stop worrying, adults. Some young people actually do care about spiritual things.** The only reason this book worked was because there really are young people out there who take their faith seriously. This faith is not just a Sunday morning thing: it's a whole life thing. You can see this in the sheer diversity of topics covered in the book. One girl comes to grip with a childhood marked by appalling abuse. Another finds a soul mate. One guy even tells a story about – get this – an idea he thought of while in the shower! (No, it's not me, but he's undoubtedly a genius.) As a whole, these stories present a picture of the way Christian young people today are living honestly and hopefully despite their imperfections. And for me personally, these stories present a picture of what God can do with a crazy idea that hits you in the middle of your morning shower.

Forty Voices: Stories of Hope from Our Generation is available at www.FortyVoices.com

summing it all up in one sentence

Originally published in *The Richmond Times Dispatch*

"Josh, I'm sorry, but we don't have any time left for you to speak."

These are not exactly the words you want to hear after you have waited all day to speak at a school awards assembly.

I could've left after my morning speech to the sophomores, but they offered to fit in five minutes for me to speak to the juniors that afternoon.

I prefer an hour, but I figured that in five minutes I could probably have an impact on at least one of the 600 people in the audience. So I decided to wait.

Big mistake.

"You mean I just waited four hours for nothing?" I demanded

"I'm really sorry about this," the assistant principle whispered to me backstage, "But we are out of time. Thanks for coming."

His right arm moved out in search of an agreeable handshake. It didn't find one.

"No, no. This is no good," I said.

"I'm sorry. There's nothing we can do."

Again, he offered a handshake, and again, I didn't give him one.

"At least let me give one sentence," I insisted. "Literally – one sentence."

He left to confer with some of his colleagues.

"OK, one sentence."

"Thank you," I said, shaking his hand.

He stepped out of the backstage area, and that was that. Only a heavy maroon curtain separated me from the 600 students in the audience as I began to nervously pace the stage, limping slightly on my artificial leg. My mind shifted into high gear as I brainstormed for that one sentence that might impact a few of the students.

It was Philosophy 101 with lots of adrenaline and no time to spare. I had one sentence to bring my seventeen years to 600 of my peers. One sentence to somehow sum up everything I felt was important.

What *was* important in life?

I went through everything I could think of. Love. Impact. God. Goals. Education. Laughter. It was the quintessence of the "main point speech." There was no time for rapport, entertainment or trust-building. It was one sentence – no more, no less. This was not a speech. This was an epitaph.

It's the question of the enduring legacy. Usually, we create our legacy by the day-to-day decisions about how we want to spend our time. But there are occasional moments of truth, those last words before we head off into a new season of life.

Like ending a monthly column you've written for the last two years.

Big decisions are tough. You want to keep doing the things you enjoy, but you want to be focused. I'm going to college next month. I've always been a believer in doing everything you can do with your abilities, but I'm an even bigger believer in focusing all you can on your primary objectives. As a student, I want to be a student. Not a student/columnist, or a student/writer, just a student.

But the decisions get harder. If you are going to leave, what do you leave behind? What do you say in that final column, to all those readers who have shared your high school days with you like a second family? And what do you leave with the 600 high school students with whom you can only share one sentence?

"Well, we have a quick speech for you," I heard someone say. "So, um, here's Josh Sundquist."

About three people clapped.

I burst out from behind the curtain, half-angry, half-excited and half-ready to scream with passion. Once I had their attention, I threw out my sentence with every bit of energy I could. Even as I spoke the words, I could feel a tingle down my spine.

"Love God, live for others and *make your life count for something!*"

exclusive offer for readers

Congratulations on finishing this book. (If you haven't finished it yet, then why are you skipping to the end? Are you the kind of person that likes to ruin movie endings for everyone else[*]?)

Good news. As a reader of *A Leg Up,* you can get exclusive access to all this stuff—free!

1. Watch the original "Fast Food Drive Thru Pranks" video Josh writes about on page 77

2. Download a copy of Josh's humor column "Will she holla back? Problems with Dating in the Modern Era," which received national acclaim in *Current, Newsweek's* college magazine

3. Enjoyed the stories in this book? Get an inspirational message from Josh each month with Josh's free e-newsletter!

Get this stuff right now at:
www.JoshSundquist.com/SpecialOffer
A Leg Up Reader Password: E2893S

---

[*] Bruce Willis is a ghost. Kevin Spacey is Kieser Sosan. Brad Pitt is imaginary. Darth Vadar is Luke's father.

acknowledgements

Thanks to my wonderful Mother for saving all of these columns over the years. This book would not have been possible without her careful scrapbooking and greatly exaggerated view of my writing skill. I love you, Mom.

Thanks to Ms. Penton for her acerbic wit that made newspaper class such a good time in high school. Also, thanks for suggesting to my Mom that she catalogue my columns and for giving me my first real platform for writing. And I appreciate you nominating me for whatever award that was that I won.

Thanks to Penelope, who allowed me the chance of a lifetime: My very own column in the *Richmond Times Dispatch* while I was still in high school. Wow. That was really cool. Thanks! And thanks for helping me get permission for these reprints.

Speaking of which, thank you to Charles Saunders at the *RTD* for arranging for reprint permission.

I would be greatly remiss if I did not acknowledge the tireless work of my assistant, Pebbles, who put large amounts of time and energy into helping compile this book. Thanks a million, Pebbles! Couldn't have done it without you.

And of course, a big shout-out to everyone in Ms. Penton's class to who helped with the compilation: Phillip Bannister, Brandon Bovia, Simona Byler, Sofia Cabrera, Savanna Cary, Lindsey Cockburn, Matt Detrow, Natalie Diehl, Alison Domonoske, Britany Fulk, Priscilla Harrison, Irene Hernandez, Heather Hunter-Nickels, Irina Kukolj, Justin L'Ecuyer, Lauren Martin, Seanice Martin-Lynch, Olivia McCarty, Aidan Newcity, David Proctor, Chris Pyle, Maria Rose, and Kiya Scott. You guys rock!

And I tip my hat to Chris and Ben at FWIS for being the best book cover designers west (or east, for that matter) of the Mississippi.

Finally, I would like to thank the many people who appear in this book, including Cool Dude #2 and #3, several girls that I had crushes on, and a variety of disgruntled fast food employees. If any of you are reading this book, hopefully you aren't too annoyed.

about the author

Josh Sundquist is a Paralympic ski racer and nationally known inspirational speaker. He has been featured on CNN and in USA TODAY and has spoken to hundreds of thousands of people across the country.

Josh began speaking to groups about his experiences at age ten. He has since shared his story as a keynote speaker at schools, associations, Fortune 500 companies, and in Washington, DC at the White House. He was the second youngest person ever accepted as a Professional Member of the National Speaker's Association.

As a writer, Josh has been published in *The Washington Post, Daily Guideposts*, and *Current, Newsweek's* college magazine. In 2003 he co-authored the teen devotional book *Forty Voices: Stories of Hope from Our Generation.*

To check Josh's availability to speak to your group, visit www.JoshSundquist.com

Order *A Leg Up* in bulk and get wholesale prices! Ideal for:
- Schools to use for character development curriculum, journalism classes, or graduation memento
- Organizations to give out as a recognition award, motivational tool, or banquet keepsake
- Also can be resold as a fundraiser

Contact Discounts@LeeAndCoBooks.com